AAOS   Stephen J. Rahm, NREMT-P

Paramedic Review Manual
for National Certification

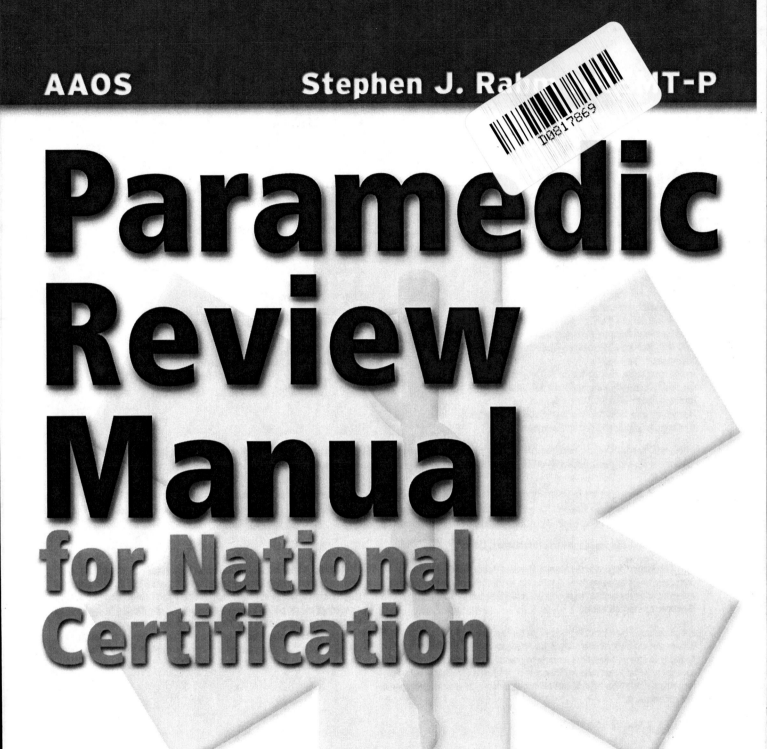

JONES AND BARTLETT PUBLISHERS

Sudbury, Massachusetts

BOSTON   TORONTO   LONDON   SINGAPORE

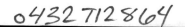

Jones and Bartlett Publishers

World Headquarters
Jones and Bartlett Publishers
40 Tall Pine Drive, Sudbury, MA 01776
978-443-5000
info@jbpub.com
www.EMSzone.com

Jones and Bartlett Publishers Canada
6339 Ormindale Way
Mississauga, ON CANADA L5V 1J2

Jones and Bartlett Publishers International
Barb House, Barb Mews
London W6 7PA, UK

Production Credits
Chief Executive Officer: Clayton E. Jones
Chief Operating Officer: Donald W. Jones, Jr.
President, Higher Education and
   Professional Publishing: Robert Holland
V.P. Sales and Marketing: William J. Kane
V.P. Production and Design: Anne Spencer
V.P. Manufacturing and Inventory Control: Therese Connell
Publisher, Public Safety Group: Kimberly Brophy
Editor: Jennifer Reed
Senior Production Editor: Linda S. DeBruyn
Senior Marketing Manager: Alisha Weisman
Text and Cover Design: Anne Spencer
Typesetting and Editorial: Carlisle Publishers Services
Printing and Binding: Courier Company

Jones and Bartlett's books and products are available through most bookstores and online booksellers. To contact Jones and Bartlett Publishers directly, call 800-832-0034, fax 978-443-8000, or visit our website, www.jbpub.com.

Substantial discounts on bulk quantities of Jones and Bartlett's publications are available to corporations, professional associations, and other qualified organizations. For details and specific discount information, contact the special sales department at Jones and Bartlett via the above contact information or send an email to specialsales@jbpub.com.

ISBN-13: 978-0-7637-5518-8

Library of Congress Cataloging in-Publication Data
Rahm, Stephen J.
   Paramedic review manual for national certification / Stephen J. Rahm; American Academy of Orthopaedic Surgeons.
     p. cm.
   ISBN 0-7637-1831-9
   1. Emergency medical technicians—Examinations, questions, etc. I. Title.
   [DNLM: 1. Emergency Medical Services—Examination Questions. 2. Emergency
Medical Technicians—Examination Questions. 3. First Aid—Examination Questions.
WX18.2 R147n 2003]
RC86.9 .R347 2003
616.02'5'076—dc21
6048
Printed in the United States of America
15 14 13 12 11   10 9 8 7 6

2002034056

Contents

Acknowledgments

Jones and Bartlett Publishers and the author would like to thank the following individuals for their time, expertise, and assistance with this series.

Michael T. Czarnecki
Brooklyn, NY

Jonathan Epstien
Needham, MA

Diane Moore
Ft. Gordon, GA

Steve Carrier
White River Junction, VT

ADDITIONAL CREDITS

Unless otherwise indicated, photographs and illustrations have been supplied by the American Academy of Orthopaedic Surgeons, Jones and Bartlett Publishers, Stephen J. Rahm, and the Maryland Institute of Emergency Medical Services System.

Section Opener 2
© Jeff Havlik/911 Pictures

Section Opener 3, Skill Station 1
© Eddie Sperling

--- **Dedication** ---

This publication is dedicated to my wife Faith because she continuously supported me throughout the development of this manual, took care of our two children, and selflessly put aside her own activities as I secluded myself behind the computer. For this and innumerable other reasons, I will forever love her.

S.J.R.

Preface

This preparatory review manual has been developed to prepare you for the National EMT-Paramedic written and practical examinations. It is important to note that this manual is not an educational tool, but rather a review and assessment of your baseline knowledge. If utilized as intended, you will be able to identify any area(s) of weakness that you may have, thus allowing you to adjust your pre-exam studies accordingly.

No part of this preparatory review manual will guarantee success on any part of the National certification exam process. However, if used as an adjunct to regular study and practice, your chances of success are maximized.

Section I of this manual provides an overview of the 1998 EMT-Paramedic National Standard Curriculum (NSC).

Section II provides you with a series of practice written examinations that are designed to stimulate your critical thinking and problem solving skills, both of which are crucial attributes that EMS providers at all levels must possess.

Section III will review all of the skills that you are required to successfully complete during the National EMT-Paramedic practical examination. For each skill, you will find helpful information, tips, pointers, and practice scenarios designed to facilitate your progression through the practical examination.

Section IV provides answers with detailed rationales for all practice examinations and scenarios.

All information contained within this review manual is based upon the 1998 EMT-Paramedic National Standard Curriculum and the 2005 Emergency Cardiac Care (ECC) guidelines for basic and advanced cardiac life support.

For further information and resources, you can visit the following websites:
• Jones and Bartlett Publishers: www.EMSzone.com
• Emergency Care and Safety Institute: www.ECSinstitute.org
• National Registry of EMTs: www.nremt.org
• U.S. Dept. of Transportation: www.nhtsa.dot.gov

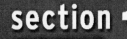

section 1

contents

The 1998 Paramedic NSC and the NREMT

The 1998 EMT-Paramedic National Standard Curriculum (NSC) will be overviewed in this section. Though the revised paramedic curriculum has increased substantially in length and depth, with the addition of several new lessons, the scope of practice of the paramedic essentially remains unchanged. The revisions made to the curriculum are intended to enhance the overall knowledge base and professional development of the paramedic.

A healthy understanding of each of the curriculum modules and knowledge objectives, coupled with adequate and effective study will greatly enhance your overall understanding of your roles, responsibilities, and duties as an EMT-Paramedic. Furthermore, frequent practice of the psychomotor skills that are addressed later in this manual will prepare you for the National EMT-Paramedic practical examination, which assesses your ability to provide safe and effective emergency medical care to patients in the field.

Refer to your paramedic textbook for the sub-objectives for each module of the paramedic curriculum. The entire 1998 EMT-Paramedic National Standard Curriculum can be downloaded from the National Highway Traffic Safety Administration (NHTSA) website at http://www.nhtsa.dot.gov.

Module 1: Preparatory

At the completion of this module, the paramedic student will understand the roles and responsibilities of a Paramedic within an EMS system, apply the basic concepts of development, pathophysiology and pharmacology to assessment and management of emergency patients, be able to properly administer medications, and communicate effectively with patients.

1-1 Understand the paramedic's roles and responsibilities within an EMS system, and how these roles and responsibilities differ from other levels of providers.

1-2 Understand and value the importance of personal wellness in EMS and serve as a healthy role model for peers.

1-3 Integrate the implementation of primary injury prevention activities as an effective way to reduce death, disabilities and health care costs.

1-4 Understand the legal issues that impact decisions made in the out-of-hospital environment.

1-5 Understand the role that ethics plays in decision-making in the out-of-hospital environment.

1-6 Apply the general concepts of pathophysiology for the assessment and management of emergency patients.

1-7 Integrate pathophysiological principles of pharmacology and the assessment findings to formulate a field impression and implement a pharmacologic management plan.

1-8 Safely and precisely access the venous circulation and administer medications.

1-9 Integrate the principles of therapeutic communication to effectively communicate with any patient while providing care.

1-10 Integrate the physiological, psychological, and sociological changes throughout human development with assessment and communication strategies for patients of all ages.

Module 2: Airway

At the completion of this module, the paramedic student will be able to establish and/ or maintain a patent airway, oxygenate, and ventilate a patient.

2-1 Establish and/ or maintain a patent airway, oxygenate, and ventilate a patient.

Module 3: Patient Assessment

At the completion of this module, the paramedic student will be able to take a proper history and perform a comprehensive physical exam on any patient, and communicate the findings to others.

3-1 Use the appropriate techniques to obtain a medical history from a patient.

3-2 Explain the pathophysiological significance of physical exam findings.

3-3 Integrate the principles of history taking and techniques of physical exam to perform a patient assessment.

3-4 Apply a process of clinical decision making to use the assessment findings to help form a field impression.

3-5 Follow an accepted format for dissemination of patient information in verbal form, either in person or over the radio.

3-6 Effectively document the essential elements of patient assessment, care and transport.

Module 4: Trauma

At the completion of this module, the paramedic student will be able to integrate pathophysiological principles and assessment findings to formulate a field impression and implement the treatment plan for the trauma patient.

4-1 Integrate the principles of kinematics to enhance the patient assessment and predict the likelihood of injuries based on the patient's mechanism of injury.

4-2 Integrate pathophysiological principles and assessment findings to formulate a field impression and implement the treatment plan for the patient with shock or hemorrhage.

4-3 Integrate pathophysiological principles and the assessment findings to formulate a field impression and implement the treatment plan for the patient with soft tissue trauma.

4-4 Integrate pathophysiological principles and the assessment findings to formulate a field impression and implement the management plan for the patient with a burn injury.

4-5 Integrate pathophysiological principles and the assessment findings to formulate a field impression and implement a treatment plan for the trauma patient with a suspected head injury.

4-6 Integrate pathophysiological principles and the assessment findings to formulate a field impression and implement a treatment plan for the patient with a suspected spinal injury.

4-7 Integrate pathophysiological principles and the assessment findings to formulate a field impression and implement a treatment plan for a patient with a thoracic injury.

4-8 Integrate pathophysiological principles and the assessment findings to formulate a field impression and implement the treatment plan for the patient with suspected abdominal trauma.

4-9 Integrate pathophysiological principles and the assessment findings to formulate a field impression and implement the treatment plan for the patient with a musculoskeletal injury.

Module 5: Medical

At the completion of this unit, the paramedic student will be able to integrate pathophysiological principles and assessment findings to formulate a field impression and implement the treatment plan for the medical patient.

5-1 Integrate pathophysiological principles and assessment findings to formulate a field impression and implement the treatment plan for the patient with respiratory problems.

5-2 Integrate pathophysiological principles and assessment findings to formulate a field impression and implement the treatment plan for the patient with cardiovascular disease.

5-3 Integrate pathophysiological principles and assessment findings to formulate a field impression and implement the treatment plan for the patient with a neurological problem.

5-4 Integrate pathophysiological principles and assessment findings to formulate a field impression and implement a treatment plan for the patient with an endocrine problem.

Module 5: Medical, continued

5-5 Integrate pathophysiological principles and assessment findings to formulate a field impression and implement a treatment plan for the patient with an allergic or anaphylactic reaction.

5-6 Integrate pathophysiological principles and assessment findings to formulate a field impression and implement the treatment plan for the patient with a gastroenterologic problem.

5-7 Integrate pathophysiological principles and the assessment findings to formulate a field impression and implement a treatment plan for the patient with a renal or urologic problem.

5-8 Integrate pathophysiological principles and assessment findings to formulate a field impression and implement a treatment plan for the patient with a toxic exposure.

5-9 Integrate the pathophysiological principles of the hematopoietic system to formulate a field impression and implement a treatment plan.

5-10 Integrate pathophysiological principles and assessment findings to formulate a field impression and implement the treatment plan for the patient with an environmentally induced or exacerbated medical or traumatic condition.

5-11 Integrate pathophysiological principles and assessment findings to formulate a field impression and implement a management plan for the patient with infectious and communicable diseases.

5-12 Describe and demonstrate safe, empathetic competence in caring for patients with behavioral emergencies.

5-13 Utilize gynecological principles and assessment findings to formulate a field impression and implement the management plan for the patient experiencing a gynecological emergency.

5-14 Apply an understanding of the anatomy and physiology of the female reproductive system to the assessment and management of a patient experiencing normal or abnormal labor.

Module 6: Special Considerations

At the completion of this unit, the paramedic student will be able to integrate pathophysiological principles and assessment findings to formulate a field impression and implement the treatment plan for neonatal, pediatric, and geriatric patients, diverse patients, and chronically ill patients.

6-1 Integrate pathophysiological principles and assessment findings to formulate a field impression and implement the treatment plan for the neonatal patient.

6-2 Integrate pathophysiological principles and assessment findings to formulate a field impression and implement the treatment plan for the pediatric patient.

6-3 Integrate the pathophysiological principles and the assessment findings to formulate and implement a treatment plan for the geriatric patient.

6-4 Integrate the assessment findings to formulate a field impression and implement a treatment plan for the patient who has sustained abuse or assault.

6-5 Integrate pathophysiological and psychosocial principles to adapt the assessment and treatment plan for diverse patients and those who face physical, mental, social and financial challenges.

6-6 Integrate the pathophysiological principles and the assessment findings to formulate a field impression and implement a treatment plan for the acute deterioration of a chronic care patient.

Module 7: Assessment-Based Management

At the completion of this unit, the paramedic student will be able to integrate pathophysiological principles and assessment findings to formulate a field impression and implement the treatment plan for patients with common complaints.

7-1 Integrate the principles of assessment-based management to perform an appropriate assessment and implement the management plan for patients with common complaints.

Module 8: Operations

At the completion of this unit, the paramedic student will be able to safely manage the scene of an emergency.

8-1 Understand standards and guidelines that help ensure safe and effective ground and air medical transport.

8-2 Integrate the principles of general incident management and multiple casualty incident (MCI) management techniques in order to function effectively at major incidents.

8-3 Integrate the principles of rescue awareness and operations to safely rescue a patient from water, hazardous atmospheres, trenches, highways, and hazardous terrain.

8-4 Evaluate hazardous materials emergencies, call for appropriate resources, and work in the cold zone.

8-5 Have an awareness of the human hazard of crime and violence and the safe operation at crime scenes and other emergencies.

In preparing for the NREMT-Paramedic written examination, it is important to have a basic understanding of the National Registry written examination process. This portion of Section I will overview the following:

- The NREMT-Paramedic test plan.
- The National EMS Practice Analysis

The NREMT-Paramedic test plan lists the six subtests that comprise the written examination and the range of items that appear on the examination for each individual subtest.

NREMT-Paramedic Test Plan

Topic	Range of # Items
1. Airway and Breathing	30–36
2. Cardiology	29–35
3. Trauma	27–33
4. Medical	24–30
5. Obstetrics and Pediatrics	25–31
6. Operations	27–33
TOTAL	180

A crucial part of this section is the National EMS Practice Analysis, which is conducted by the NREMT. The NREMT written examinations reflect subject matter-identified as being critical tasks-that is extrapolated from the practice analysis.

The purpose of the National EMS Practice Analysis is to identify the following information:

- The tasks most frequently performed by paramedics in the field.
- The criticality of the tasks with regard to the overall outcome of the patient.
- The potential for harm if the tasks were performed both correctly and incorrectly.

With the above information identified, the NREMT is able to develop written examinations that accurately reflect the care provided by the paramedics. Successful completion of the NREMT-Paramedic written and practical examination process serves as formal verification of entry-level competence in providing safe and effective emergency medical care.

To ensure an accurate reflection of EMS care in the field, the NREMT conducts the practice analysis every 5 years. Regardless of the frequency with which paramedic textbooks and other publications are revised, the NREMT-Paramedic written examination is based on the most current practice analysis.

All levels of the NREMT written examination are based upon the same critical tasks identified in the practice analysis. The only difference is the level of knowledge required based on the examination being taken (ie, EMT-B versus paramedic).

The NREMT examination items are developed to measure the important tasks of practice as an emergency care provider. Items are drafted in relationship to the tasks identified by a committee of National EMS experts that relate directly to the job of a provider. The domain of practice that limits therapy in an item is based upon national standard curricula developed by the National Highway Traffic Safety Administration. The tasks included in the practice analysis were presented to EMS providers in the form of a survey. The providers, by their responses, inform the NREMT of the frequency, criticality, and difficulty in performing an identified task. This data is then analyzed and a report, "The National EMS Practice Analysis" defines the important tasks involved in the occupations of being an EMS provider at one of the various levels of care. EMS educational programs are encouraged to review the practice analysis when teaching courses and as part of the final review of the abilities of the students to perform the tasks required for competent practice.

Practice Exams

This section contains seven practice exams totaling 360 questions. The first six exams contain 30 questions each and represent the individual subtests that comprise the National EMT-Paramedic written examination. You should focus your preparatory studies in any area(s) that you answered nine or more questions incorrectly.

Following the individual subtests, you will take a comprehensive 180-item final practice exam, which reflects all six subtests in a scrambled fashion. At the end of the final practice exam, you will find a blueprint that categorizes each question into a subtest area and suggests a minimum number of correctly answered questions.

In order to obtain a reliable assessment of your baseline knowledge, it is highly recommended that you complete each individual test in its entirety prior to reading the correct answers and detailed rationales, which can be found in Section IV of this manual.

All practice questions in this section are based upon the following:
• 1998 EMT-Paramedic National Standard Curriculum
• 2005 Emergency Cardiac Care (ECC) guidelines and algorithms
• 2004 Brain Trauma Foundation (BTF) guidelines

Subtest 1 Practice Exam: Airway and Breathing

_____ **1.** Which of the following signs would indicate inadequate breathing in a 42-year-old man?
 a. Expiratory wheezing and pink, moist skin
 b. Respirations at a rate of 18 breaths/min with reduced tidal volume
 c. Eupneic respirations at a rate of 26 breaths/min
 d. Audible rhonchi and flushed skin

_____ **2.** What is the BEST airway device to use in a deeply unconscious intoxicated patient?
 a. Oropharyngeal airway
 b. Nasopharyngeal airway
 c. Endotracheal tube
 d. Laryngeal mask airway

_____ **3.** You have intubated a 33-year-old woman in cardiac arrest secondary to trauma. During your 5-point auscultation, you note an absence of breath sounds in the right hemithorax. What does this finding MOST likely indicate?
 a. Left mainstem bronchus intubation
 b. Intubation of the hypopharyngeal area
 c. Potential internal injury to the thorax
 d. Inadvertent intubation of the esophagus

_____ **4.** Immediately after placing an endotracheal tube in an adult patient, the paramedic should
 a. attach a BVM device and ventilate.
 b. attach an end-tidal carbon dioxide detector.
 c. inflate the distal cuff with 5 to 10 mL of air.
 d. auscultate over the lungs and epigastrium.

_____ **5.** A 56-year-old woman calls EMS because of a sudden onset of difficulty breathing. When you assess her, you note that she is only able to speak in two-word sentences. Your initial management should include
 a. positive pressure ventilations with 100% oxygen.
 b. supplemental oxygen through a nonrebreathing mask.
 c. immediate nasotracheal intubation.
 d. determining the cause of her problem.

_____ **6.** Which of the following signs is LEAST reliable when assessing the ventilatory status of an adult patient?
 a. Chest wall excursion
 b. Distal capillary refill
 c. State of alertness
 d. Breath sounds

_____ **7.** A 21-year-old man is semiconscious and has shallow, gurgling respirations. After opening the airway, the paramedic should
 a. begin assisting ventilations.
 b. suction the oropharynx.
 c. prepare for intubation.
 d. attach a pulse oximeter.

_____ **8.** Snoring respirations in an elderly woman found unconscious in her bed are MOST rapidly managed by
   a. inserting a simple airway adjunct.
   b. manually maneuvering the head.
   c. suctioning of the oropharynx.
   d. performing a digital intubation.

_____ **9.** Which of the following signs would be MOST indicative of an upper airway obstruction?
   a. Anxiety and a forceful cough
   b. Flushed skin and tachycardia
   c. Confusion and low oxygen saturation
   d. Ability to speak in broken sentences

_____ **10.** Which of the following clinical signs is MOST indicative of *adequate* breathing?
   a. Reduced tidal volume
   b. Tachypnea and hypopnea
   c. Pink oral mucous membranes
   d. Unilateral chest wall movement

━━━━━ **Questions 11–13 apply to the following scenario** ━━━━━
You are called to the home of an elderly woman who reports respiratory distress. The patient is awake and alert and is able to easily answer your questions. She has a blood pressure of 160/90 mm Hg, an irregular pulse rate of 110 beats/min, and slightly labored respirations of 26 breaths/min. As you further assess the patient, you note the presence of perioral cyanosis.

_____ **11.** On the basis of this information, the paramedic's initial approach to management should include
   a. applying a nasal cannula at 4 to 6 L/min.
   b. applying a nonrebreathing mask at 15 L/min.
   c. initiating some form of positive pressure ventilation.
   d. sedating the patient and performing intubation.

_____ **12.** Which of the following would occur if the patient's respirations became shallow and increased to a rate of 32 breaths/min?
   a. The tidal volume would increase.
   b. The minute volume would remain unchanged.
   c. The tidal volume and minute volume would remain unchanged.
   d. An increase in the amount of dead space air would develop.

_____ **13.** The patient has a respiratory rate of 26 breaths/min. On the basis of her chest rise, you estimate her tidal volume to be approximately 450 mL. What is her approximate alveolar minute volume?
   a. 8,200 mL
   b. 9,400 mL
   c. 10,100 mL
   d. 11,700 mL

_____ **14.** You are ventilating a patient with a BVM device and note minimal rise of the chest with each ventilation. What should your initial course of action be?
   a. Check for damage to the BVM device.
   b. Reposition the patient's head as needed.
   c. Switch to a pocket face mask with oxygen.
   d. Suction the patient's oropharynx for 15 seconds.

_____ **15.** You are assisting ventilations of a 40-year-old male with a BVM. The patient is semiconscious and has a heart rate of 140 beats/min. Which of the following signs would indicate that your assisted ventilations are *inadequate*?
   a. Equal chest wall excursion
   b. Minimal abdominal movement
   c. A marked increase in heart rate
   d. Increased ventilation compliance

_____ **16.** Which of the following statements regarding end-tidal CO_2 ($ETCO_2$) monitoring following endotracheal intubation is MOST correct?
   a. $ETCO_2$ monitoring is most reliable in patients with poor pulmonary perfusion
   b. The $ETCO_2$ detector is not affected by endotracheally administered medications
   c. $ETCO_2$ monitoring is superior to all methods of confirming proper tube placement
   d. $ETCO_2$ monitoring should be used in conjunction with a careful clinical assessment

_____ **17.** A 20-year-old male presents with signs of a mild upper airway obstruction. He is conscious, anxious, and coughing forcefully. You should
   a. insert a nasopharyngeal airway to maintain airway patency.
   b. perform laryngoscopy and remove the obstruction with Magill forceps.
   c. perform subdiaphragmatic thrusts with the patient in a standing position.
   d. closely monitor the patient's condition and encourage him to keep coughing.

_____ **18.** Through which of the following airway devices can you achieve the greatest ventilatory volume?
   a. Nonrebreathing mask
   b. Pocket face mask
   c. BVM device
   d. BVM device with an oral airway

_____ **19.** Following intubation of a patient in respiratory arrest, you are able to hear clear, equal breath sounds bilaterally and audible epigastric sounds. What is the next step in management?
   a. Inflate the distal cuff with 5 to 10 mL of air.
   b. Withdraw the tube approximately 1 to 2 cm.
   c. Remove the tube and hyperoxygenate the patient.
   d. Secure the tube and resume ventilations.

_____**20.** What is the MOST appropriate initial action for the paramedic to take when a previously breathing patient suddenly becomes apneic?
   a. Evaluate for breathing for 30 seconds.
   b. Assess for the presence of a pulse.
   c. Initiate positive pressure ventilations.
   d. Perform endotracheal intubation.

_____ **21.** In a normal healthy individual, breathing is primarily stimulated by
   a. an increase in arterial CO_2.
   b. an increase in arterial O_2.
   c. a decrease in arterial O_2.
   d. a decrease in arterial CO_2.

_____**22.** Management of an unconscious patient with respirations of 14 breaths/min and adequate tidal volume should consist of
   a. performing immediate intubation to protect the patient's airway.
   b. inserting an airway adjunct and providing assisted ventilations.
   c. inserting an airway adjunct and providing oxygen through a nonrebreathing mask.
   d. inserting an airway adjunct and suctioning the mouth every 30 seconds.

_____**23.** When ventilating an adult cardiac arrest patient via the ET tube, you should:
   a. deliver each breath over a period of 2 seconds at a rate of 20 breaths/min.
   b. instruct the compressor to stop compressions while you deliver ventilations.
   c. deliver each breath over a period of 1 second at a rate of 8 to 10 breaths/min.
   d. instruct the compressor to continue compressions as you hyperventilate the patient.

_____**24.** You are ventilating a severely dehydrated apneic 70-year-old male with a history of end-stage emphysema. In order to minimize the risk of lowering the patient's cardiac output and blood pressure, you should
   a. use a manually-triggered ventilation device.
   b. hyperventilate the patient at 20 to 24 breaths/min.
   c. adjust the ventilation rate to allow complete exhalation.
   d. use a device that provides positive-end expiratory pressure.

_____ **25.** You are administering supplemental oxygen to a conscious patient with a nonrebreathing mask when he suddenly pulls the mask from his face. You should
   a. increase the flow rate and replace the mask.
   b. securely tape the mask to the patient's face.
   c. apply a nasal cannula at 2 to 6 L/min.
   d. offer the patient a simple face mask instead.

_____**26.** An unconscious, apneic patient has sustained massive facial trauma including a mandibular fracture and severe oral bleeding. Intubation has been attempted without success. What form of airway management should be taken next?
   a. Digital intubation
   b. Blind nasotracheal intubation
   c. BVM device ventilations with 100% oxygen
   d. Needle or surgical cricothyroidotomy

_____ **27.** Prior to applying a nonrebreathing mask on a conscious patient with respiratory distress, you should
- **a.** ensure that the reservoir bag is fully inflated.
- **b.** set the oxygen flowmeter to no more than 10 L/min.
- **c.** ask the patient to exhale fully and then hold his breath.
- **d.** place the patient in the recovery position in the event of vomiting.

────── **Questions 28–30 apply to the following scenario** ──────

You and your paramedic partner are standing by at the scene of a structural fire when one of the firefighters approaches you in obvious respiratory distress. He states that he entered the structure without a self-contained breathing apparatus and was exposed to a significant amount of smoke. He is awake, alert, and in moderate respiratory distress. You obtain vital signs that show a blood pressure of 156/90 mm Hg, a strong pulse rate of 120 beats/min, and labored respirations of 28 breaths/min. The pulse oximeter shows a reading of 93%.

_____ **28.** Initial airway management for this patient should include
- **a.** a nasal cannula at 6 L/min.
- **b.** a simple face mask at 10 L/min.
- **c.** a nonrebreathing mask at 15 L/min.
- **d.** assisted ventilations with a BVM device.

_____ **29.** As your partner is gathering information for the patient care report, you note that the patient's level of consciousness has markedly decreased. Additionally, you can hear loud stridor on inhalation and the pulse oximeter now reads 85%. What should be your FIRST course of action?
- **a.** Ensure that you are delivering humidified oxygen.
- **b.** Perform immediate intubation before the airway closes.
- **c.** Perform an emergency needle cricothyroidotomy.
- **d.** Provide assisted ventilations and prepare for intubation.

_____ **30.** In managing this patient, you use a capnographer. What information will this device provide?
- **a.** Oxygen saturation level
- **b.** Amount of exhaled carbon dioxide
- **c.** Residual level of oxygen in the lungs
- **d.** Percentage of functional alveoli in the lungs

Subtest 2 Practice Exam: Cardiology

_____ **1.** Chest pain of cardiac origin is MOST commonly described by the patient as
- **a.** sharp.
- **b.** stabbing.
- **c.** crushing.
- **d.** cramping.

A patient with a crushing chest pain displays the rhythm shown below:

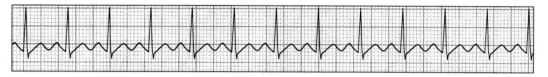

_____ 2. What is the MOST detrimental effect that the above rhythm can have on this patient?
   a. Increased nervousness and anxiety
   b. Decreased myocardial irritability
   c. Decreased myocardial contractility
   d. Increased myocardial oxygen demand

_____ 3. Which of the following signs or symptoms is LEAST suggestive of cardiac compromise?
   a. Tachypnea
   b. Cephalgia
   c. Orthopnea
   d. Tachycardia

_____ 4. Cardiopulmonary arrest in the adult population is MOST often secondary to
   a. acute myocardial infarction.
   b. cardiac arrhythmia.
   c. massive hypovolemia.
   d. accidental electrocution.

─────── **Questions 5-7 pertain to the following scenario:** ───────

A 57-year-old man reports dull pain in his chest. He tells you that he has had two heart attacks within the past 3 years and is currently being treated for hypertension. His medications include digoxin, diltiazem hydrochloride, and a "water pill." He has a blood pressure of 166/90 mm Hg, a pulse rate of 112 beats/min, and respirations of 22 breaths/min.

_____ 5. As your partner is preparing to administer 100% to the patient, you should
   a. obtain a 12-lead ECG tracing.
   b. administer up to 325 mg of aspirin.
   c. start an IV line of normal saline.
   d. administer up to 3 doses of nitroglycerin.

The patient is displaying the cardiac rhythm shown below:

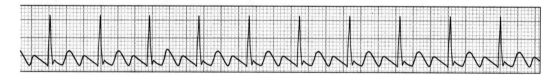

_____ 6. You should interpret the above cardiac rhythm as
   a. atrial flutter with a fixed block.
   b. atrial flutter with a variable block.
   c. uncontrolled atrial fibrillation.
   d. second-degree AV block type II.

_____ **7.** The MOST appropriate management for the above rhythm should consist of
a. sedation and synchronized cardioversion.
b. 150 mg of amiodarone given over 10 minutes.
c. close monitoring and transport to the hospital.
d. 0.25 mg/kg of diltiazem given over 2 minutes.

_____ **8.** Secondary ventricular fibrillation would be caused by all of the following conditions, EXCEPT
a. acute myocardial infarction.
b. massive pulmonary embolism.
c. a sudden cardiac arrhythmia.
d. a ruptured cerebral aneurysm.

_____ **9.** You are called to the home of a 60-year-old woman who has had chest pressure for the past 48 hours. At present, she is conscious but extremely weak. She has a blood pressure of 80/40 mm Hg, a thready pulse rate of 120 beats/min, and slightly shallow respirations of 24 breaths/min. The cardiac monitor is displaying a sinus tachycardia with marked ST segment elevation. After you place her on 100% oxygen and initiate an IV line, you should next
a. initiate a 5 to10 μg/kg/min infusion of dopamine.
b. administer a 250 to 500 mL bolus of normal saline solution.
c. administer 0.4 mg of nitroglycerin sublingually.
d. administer 2 to 4 mg of morphine by slow IV push.

_____ **10.** An elderly man is suddenly awakened in the middle of the night "gasping for air." On your arrival, you note that he is extremely restless and pale. Additionally, you see small amounts of dried blood on his lips. On the basis of this information, what is your initial field impression?
a. Unstable angina pectoris
b. Upper gastrointestinal bleed
c. Left side heart failure
d. Right side heart failure

You are transporting a 39-year-old man with a possible acute myocardial infarction to the hospital when he suddenly loses consciousness. You glance at the cardiac monitor and observe the following rhythm:

_____ **11.** After establishing that the patient is pulseless and apneic, your FIRST action should be to
a. deliver an immediate precordial thump.
b. begin CPR for 1 minute, then defibrillate.
c. increase the gain sensitivity on the cardiac monitor.
d. administer 1 mg of epinephrine by rapid IV push.

_____ **12.** All of the following medications are appropriate to administer to adult patients with asystole EXCEPT
a. 1 mg of atropine.
b. 1 mg/kg of lidocaine.
c. 1 mg of epinephrine.
d. 40 units of vasopressin.

_____ **13.** You are assessing a 50-year-old man with acute epigastric discomfort, diaphoresis, and nausea. The 12-lead ECG tracing reveals 3-mm ST segment elevation in leads II, III, and aVF. This finding is MOST consistent with
a. injury to the inferior myocardial wall.
b. ischemia of the lateral myocardial wall.
c. injury to the anterior myocardial wall.
d. ischemia of the posterior myocardial wall.

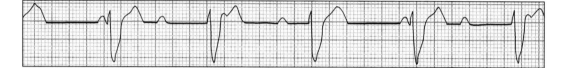

_____ **14.** You should interpret the above cardiac rhythm as
a. first-degree AV block.
b. second-degree AV block type I.
c. second-degree AV block type II.
d. third-degree AV block.

_____ **15.** Which of the following statements is FALSE regarding the automated external defibrillator (AED)?
a. A dose-attenuating system should be used with the AED in children
b. The AED should be applied to all patients at risk for cardiac arrest
c. AEDs have a high specificity for recognizing shockable cardiac rhythms
d. The AED will not analyze the cardiac rhythm if it detects patient movement

_____ **16.** You have defibrillated a patient in ventricular fibrillation and note a rhythm change to a wide complex tachycardia. What should you do next?
a. Cardiovert at 360 joules.
b. Administer an antiarrhythmic.
c. Evaluate the patient's airway.
d. Assess for a carotid pulse.

_____ **17.** Nitroglycerin is given to patients with suspected cardiac chest pain because of its physiologic effects of smooth muscle
a. contraction and increased afterload.
b. contraction and decreased preload.
c. relaxation and decreased preload.
d. relaxation and increased preload.

_____ **18.** Which of the following represents the correct dosing regimen of adenosine for a patient with a narrow complex tachycardia?
   a. 6 mg, followed by 12 mg repeated once
   b. 6 mg, followed by 12 mg repeated twice
   c. A total of 36 mg in three 12-mg increments
   d. An initial dose of 12 mg, followed by 24 mg

_____ **19.** Your patient is a 30-year-old man who had one episode of vomiting shortly after his morning workout at the gym. He is awake and alert and states that he has a slight headache. He denies chest pain or shortness of breath. Vital signs show a blood pressure of 138/68 mm Hg, a pulse rate of 42 beats/min, and respirations of 18 breaths/min. The MOST appropriate management for this patient includes
   a. IV administration of 0.5 mg atropine sulfate and oxygen.
   b. 2 to 10 μg/min infusion of epinephrine.
   c. 6 mg of adenosine, followed by a bolus of normal saline solution.
   d. supportive care and transport to the hospital.

_____ **20.** Which of the following BEST describes the appropriate questioning technique when inquiring about a patient's chest pain?
   a. Does the pain radiate to your jaw?
   b. Is the pain in the center of your chest?
   c. Can you describe the pain?
   d. Is the pain sharp or dull?

_____ **21.** Which of the following signs/symptoms would MOST likely indicate angina pectoris as opposed to an acute myocardial infarction?
   a. Normal electrocardiogram findings
   b. Presence of dyspnea
   c. Pain that lasts more than 15 minutes
   d. Pain that occurs with exertion

_____ **22.** You have just performed a synchronized cardioversion on an unstable patient with a narrow complex tachycardia. You glance at the monitor and see coarse ventricular fibrillation. The patient is pulseless and apneic. What is the next step in management?
   a. Immediately defibrillate with 360 joules.
   b. Start CPR and prepare to intubate the patient.
   c. Turn off the synchronize mode and defibrillate.
   d. Administer 100 mg of lidocaine by IV push.

_____ **23.** You are unable to obtain IV access or intubate a patient who is in cardiac arrest. The monitor shows ventricular fibrillation. What is the best course of action?
   a. Wait until drug access is available and then defibrillate.
   b. Continue CPR with basic airway management while en route to the hospital.
   c. Administer vasopressin directly into the antecubital vein.
   d. Defibrillate once at 360 joules and immediately resume CPR.

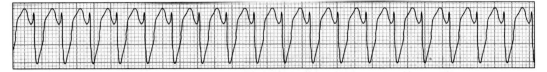

_____ **24.** You are transporting a 44-year-old man with chest pain when the above rhythm develops. The patient becomes diaphoretic and has a blood pressure of 80/60 mm Hg. The MOST appropriate management should include
a. 150 mg of amiodarone over 10 minutes.
b. 20 to 50 mg/min of procainamide hydrochloride.
c. cardioversion at 100 joules.
d. defibrillation at 200 joules.

_____ **25.** The recommended treatment sequence for a patient with a regular cardiac rhythm at a rate of 50 beats/min and no pulse includes
a. intubation or IV, CPR, and epinephrine.
b. intubation or IV, CPR, and atropine sulfate.
c. CPR, intubation or IV, epinephrine, and atropine sulfate.
d. CPR, intubation or IV, atropine, and transcutaneous pacing.

_____ **26.** Which of the following causes of pulseless electrical activity (PEA) would be MOST likely to respond to treatment in the field?
a. Hypokalemia
b. Hypovolemia
c. Lactic acidosis
d. Coronary thrombosis

_____ **27.** Following resuscitation of a patient into a perfusing rhythm, the paramedic should immediately
a. begin an antiarrhythmic infusion.
b. obtain the patient's blood pressure.
c. provide a bolus of normal saline solution.
d. reassess the patient's airway status.

_____ **28.** A 145-pound man requires a dopamine infusion at 15 μg/kg/min for severe hypotension. You have a premixed bag containing 800 mg of dopamine in 500 mL of normal saline. If you are using a microdrip administration set (60 gtts/mL), how many drops per minute should you deliver to achieve the required dose?
a. 30
b. 36
c. 42
d. 48

_____ **29.** You are treating a patient with ventricular fibrillation. As the defibrillator is charging, you should
a. visually confirm that nobody is touching the patient.
b. ask your partner to ventilate the patient at 20 breaths/min.
c. check the defibrillator to ensure the synchronizer is activated.
d. ensure that CPR is continuing until the defibrillator is charged.

_____ **30.** In which of the following situations should transcutaneous cardiac pacing (TCP) be initiated without delay?
  a. Pulseless electrical activity at a rate of 80 beats/min.
  b. Asystole, but only after 10 minutes of effective CPR.
  c. First-degree AV block in a patient with abdominal pain.
  d. Third-degree AV block in a patient with pulmonary edema.

Subtest 3 Practice Exam: Trauma

_____ **1.** Which of the following injuries would pose the MOST immediate threat to a patient's life?
  a. Bilateral femur fractures
  b. Open pneumothorax
  c. Cerebral contusion
  d. Crushed pelvis

_____ **2.** When securing a patient with a suspected spinal injury to a long backboard, it is important to
  a. log roll the patient and secure him to the board when he is on his side.
  b. secure the head first in case the patient has a cervical fracture.
  c. secure the torso as your partner maintains manual stabilization of the head.
  d. apply heavy devices such as sandbags to provide lateral stabilization of the head.

——————— **Questions 3-5 pertain to the following scenario:**———————
A 34-year-old man who was working at a construction site fell approximately 25' and landed on his head; he was not wearing a safety helmet. When you perform your initial assessment, you note that he is semiconscious and has slow, irregular respirations. You also note that the patient has trismus and is bleeding from the nose.

_____ **3.** As your partner maintains manual stabilization of the patient's head, you should
  a. begin ventilation assistance with a BVM device and 100% oxygen.
  b. start an IV, administer Versed and Norcuron, and intubate the patient.
  c. suction the nose for 15 seconds and prepare for nasotracheal intubation.
  d. apply a nonrebreathing mask and set the flow rate at 15 liters per minute.

_____ **4.** The baseline vital signs on this patient are a blood pressure of 160/90 mm Hg, a bounding pulse rate of 76 beats/min, and deep respirations of 36 breaths/min. What set of repeat vital signs would be MOST suggestive of increased intracranial pressure?
  a. BP 80/40, pulse 68 and weak, respirations 20 and deep
  b. BP 90/60, pulse 130 and weak, respirations 34 and shallow
  c. BP 174/80, pulse 120 and thready, respirations 30 and shallow
  d. BP 180/88, pulse 64 and bounding, respirations 40 and deep

_____ **5.** What is the MOST appropriate management for this patient?
  a. Hyperventilation, fluid restriction, and rapid transport
  b. Hyperventilation, 500-mL fluid bolus, rapid transport
  c. Ventilatory assistance, 500-mL fluid bolus, rapid transport
  d. Ventilatory assistance, fluid restriction, rapid transport

_____ **6.** While performing a rapid trauma assessment on a critically injured patient, you note the presence of flat jugular veins and absent breath sounds in the right hemithorax, which is dull to percussion. What is the best course of action?

  a. Treat for shock and continue with your assessment.

  b. Perform a needle thoracentesis to the right hemithorax.

  c. Stop your assessment and immediately intubate the patient.

  d. Place the patient on his left side and continue your assessment.

_____ **7.** External bleeding is MOST difficult to control in a patient who has a laceration to the

  a. brachial artery and a systolic blood pressure of 60 mm Hg.

  b. femoral artery and a blood pressure of 160/90 mm Hg.

  c. popliteal artery and a blood pressure of 120/78 mm Hg.

  d. jugular vein and a blood pressure of 80/40 mm Hg.

_____ **8.** Immediate care for a severely burned patient includes

  a. stopping the burning process.

  b. applying dressings to the burns.

  c. moving the patient to safety.

  d. ensuring a patent airway.

_____ **9.** Using the adult Rule of Nines, what percentage of the body surface area does the anterior thorax account for?

  a. 9%

  b. 18%

  c. 27%

  d. 36%

_____ **10.** A 40-year-old patient jumped approximately 20' from the roof of his house and landed on his feet. On the basis of the mechanism of injury, you should suspect injuries to which of the following structures?

  a. Knees, pelvis, and thoracic spine

  b. Tibia/fibula, pelvis, and lumbar spine

  c. Calcaneus, hips, and cervical spine

  d. Calcaneus, hips, and lumbar spine

_____ **11.** Which of the following represents the MOST appropriate technique for performing a rapid extrication from an automobile?

  a. Apply an extrication collar, maintain manual stabilization of the head, rotate the patient onto the long spine board, and remove from the automobile.

  b. Apply an extrication collar and remove the patient from the automobile on a short spine board.

  c. Apply a vest-style extraction device and slide the patient onto a long spine board in the same position in which he was found.

  d. Maintain manual stabilization of the head without an extrication collar, grasp the patient's clothing, and remove him from the automobile.

_____ **12.** Following a spinal injury, your patient experiences a loss of proprioception. This means that
   a. the patient is unable to comprehend simple questions.
   b. the body's temperature assumes that of the environment.
   c. motor function is decreased proximal to the site of the injury.
   d. the patient is unaware of one body part in relation to another.

_____ **13.** While performing a rapid trauma assessment on the victim of a shooting, you discover an open wound to the right anterior chest. What is the MOST appropriate action?
   a. Make a mental note of the injury and proceed with the assessment.
   b. Stop your assessment and prepare for immediate transport.
   c. Take steps to prevent air from entering the chest wound.
   d. Immediately reevaluate the patency of the patient's airway.

_____ **14.** You respond to the scene of a local knife-throwing contest where a young man has a large knife impaled in the precordial area, just to the left of the lower third of the sternum. Assessment reveals that he is in full cardiac arrest. Prior to transport to the hospital, what is the best course of action?
   a. Stabilize the knife in place and initiate CPR.
   b. Carefully remove the knife, control bleeding, and initiate CPR.
   c. Stabilize the knife in place.
   d. Carefully remove the knife and attach an AED.

_____ **15.** A young woman has been involved in a motor vehicle accident and is still in her car. Among other injuries, you note that there are large volumes of bright red blood spurting from the region of her groin. After ensuring airway and breathing adequacy, you should
   a. perform immediate extrication.
   b. complete a rapid trauma assessment.
   c. apply direct pressure to the wound.
   d. administer 100% oxygen via a face mask.

_____ **16.** During your assessment of a patient with a suspected head injury, you note the presence of a pinkish fluid draining from the nose. What does this MOST likely indicate?
   a. A cribriform plate fracture
   b. A basilar skull fracture
   c. An orbital skull fracture
   d. Trauma to the sinuses

_____ **17.** While assessing a patient with a painful deformity to the left upper arm, you should
   a. evaluate the brachial artery.
   b. manipulate the injury to elicit crepitus.
   c. assess the pulse most distal to the injury.
   d. assess the pulse at the popliteal artery.

_____ **18.** Appropriate management for a patient with a closed chest injury and signs of shock includes
   a. applying and inflating the PASG.
   b. initiating one IV line at a rate of 125 mL/h.
   c. ruling out a pneumothorax with a thoracentesis.
   d. applying a cardiac monitor to assess for arrhythmias.

_____ **19.** Which of the following mechanisms of injury would be LEAST likely to require a rapid trauma assessment?
   a. A 6'2" man who fell 19' from a roof
   b. A stable patient whose friend was killed in the same car
   c. A large knife impaled in the mid thigh with controlled bleeding
   d. A small-caliber gunshot wound to the left lower abdominal quadrant

_____ **20.** When controlling severe external bleeding from an extremity, which of the following techniques is usually performed simultaneously with direct pressure?
   a. Pressure point control
   b. Elevation of the extremity
   c. Application of a pressure bandage
   d. Application of a loose tourniquet

_____ **21.** Initial care for a patient with a large bleeding avulsion to the left lower leg includes
   a. assessing a pedal pulse.
   b. splinting the entire extremity.
   c. cleaning the wound with peroxide.
   d. applying a sterile dressing to the wound.

_____ **22.** A 54-year-old man is stabbed in the abdomen in an altercation. He has a 2" loop of bowel protruding from the wound. Your first action should be to
   a. ensure airway patency.
   b. control any bleeding from the wound.
   c. apply a moist, sterile dressing to the wound.
   d. gently replace the bowel back into the wound.

_____ **23.** Which of the following signs would indicate a severe pericardial tamponade?
   a. A strengthening of the pulse during inhalation
   b. A rise in the systolic pressure and a fall in the diastolic pressure
   c. Flattened jugular veins when the patient is placed at a 45-degree angle
   d. A drop in the blood pressure of greater than 10 mm Hg during inhalation

_____ **24.** Following a motorcycle accident, examination of a 40-year-old woman reveals a deformity to the fifth and sixth thoracic vertebrae, a blood pressure of 80/50 mm Hg, and a pulse rate of 74 beats/min. You should be MOST suspicious of
   a. failure of the sympathetic nervous system.
   b. posterior pressure on the heart from spinal cord swelling.
   c. damage to the parasympathetic nervous system.
   d. spinal fracture with associated myocardial damage.

_____ **25.** General care for full-thickness burns includes
  a. covering the burns with moist, sterile dressings.
  b. irrigating the burned areas with sterile saline solution.
  c. preserving the patient's body temperature.
  d. applying an antibiotic burn cream.

_____ **26.** Which of the following assessment findings would be LEAST indicative of spinal cord injury?
  a. Priapism
  b. Posturing
  c. Paresthesia
  d. Paralysis

_____ **27.** A 30-year-old man sustains an obvious head injury. You are unable to locate any other injuries during your rapid assessment. He has a blood pressure of 98/68 mm Hg, a weak pulse rate of 118 beats/min, and respirations of 28 breaths/min. Which of the following represents the MOST appropriate management for this patient?
  a. Hyperventilation with 100% oxygen and IV fluid restriction
  b. Elevation of the head of the spine board and prevention of hyperthermia
  c. 100% oxygen and IV fluids to maintain adequate perfusion
  d. 100% oxygen and 40 mg of furosemide to decrease intracranial swelling

_____ **28.** During your rapid trauma assessment of a young man who sustained blunt trauma to the anterior chest, you note paradoxical movement to the left hemithorax. What is the next step in management?
  a. Perform an immediate needle thoracentesis.
  b. Provide hand stabilization and continue the assessment.
  c. Instruct your partner to immediately intubate the patient.
  d. Circumferentially tape the chest wall for thoracic support.

_____ **29.** Which of the following is considered the earliest sign of shock?
  a. A rapid, thready pulse
  b. Absence of peripheral pulses
  c. Weak carotid and femoral pulses
  d. Increased rate of respirations

_____ **30.** Which of the following patients is MOST in need of a rapid extrication following an automobile accident?
  a. 16-year-old girl with a laceration to her forehead and tachycardia
  b. 28-year-old man with a unilateral femur fracture and confusion
  c. 40-year-old man with an open head injury and exposed brain mater
  d. 56-year-old woman with a Colles' fracture and emotional upset

Subtest 4 Practice Exam: Medical

─────── **Questions 1 and 2 pertain to the following scenario:**───────
You are called to a nearby alley where a young woman has been found unconscious. When you arrive, a police officer greets you and states that he recognizes the patient and has arrested her before for selling illegal drugs. Examination findings include a blood pressure of 60/40 mm Hg, shallow respirations of 6 breaths/min, a pulse rate of 40 beats/min, and constricted pupils.

_____ 1. After rendering the appropriate airway management, you apply the cardiac monitor and note a sinus bradycardia. After your partner obtains IV access, you should next administer
   a. a 500-mL bolus of saline solution.
   b. 0.5 mg of atropine.
   c. 1.0 mg/kg of lidocaine.
   d. 0.4 to 2.0 mg of naloxone.

_____ 2. Which of the following findings is the MOST likely cause of the patient's hypotension?
   a. Profound hypovolemia
   b. Increased parasympathetic tone
   c. Central nervous system depression
   d. Increased ventricular irritability

_____ 3. Initial management for a patient experiencing a heat-related emergency includes
   a. administering 100% oxygen.
   b. initiating rapid cooling measures.
   c. starting an IV line.
   d. removing the patient to a cooler area.

_____ 4. Which of the following findings is MOST indicative of hyperglycemic ketoacidosis?
   a. Acute onset
   b. Hyperpnea
   c. Diaphoresis
   d. Bradypnea

_____ 5. A 43-year-old woman is stung by a scorpion. Within approximately 10 minutes, she has a generalized rash and swelling to the face. The patient is now confused and has a blood pressure of 88/66 mm Hg. Management for this patient should include oxygen and
   a. IM or SC administration of 50 to 100 mg of diphenhydramine hydrochloride.
   b. IV administration of 0.03 to 0.05 mg 1:10,000 epinephrine.
   c. IV administration of 0.3 to 0.5 mg 1:10,000 epinephrine.
   d. SC administration of 0.3 to 0.5 mg 1:1,000 epinephrine.

_____ **6.** You are called to the residence of an elderly man whose daughter states that he is not acting right. The patient becomes combative when you attempt to assess him. He refuses supplemental oxygen and states that you are not taking him anywhere. What is your MOST appropriate course of action?
   a. Use soft restraints on the patient and transport him to the hospital.
   b. Calmly talk to the patient as you attempt to obtain a glucose reading.
   c. Administer 5 mg of diazepam IM to calm the patient down.
   d. Give the patient oral glucose and instruct him to swallow the contents.

_____ **7.** Which of the following findings would be MOST indicative of an infectious or communicable disease?
   a. Persistent fever
   b. Headache with photophobia
   c. Sore throat and nasal discharge
   d. Diarrhea for 3 days

_____ **8.** You respond to a call for a domestic dispute. When you arrive, you are met by a woman who tells you that her boyfriend is upstairs with a gun. He has been depressed lately. How should this situation be managed prior to police arrival?
   a. Send the woman upstairs to attempt to reason with the man.
   b. Attempt to make contact with the patient to provide care.
   c. Wait in the ambulance until police have secured the scene.
   d. Get in the ambulance and leave the scene immediately.

_____ **9.** A 39-year-old man reports nausea, lack of coordination, and frequently recurring headaches that have been getting progressively worse over the past 2 months. He denies any past medical history. On the basis of this presentation, which of the following should you suspect?
   a. Chronic epidural hematoma
   b. Space-occupying intracranial lesion
   c. Acute subarachnoid hemorrhage
   d. Ruptured cerebral arterial aneurysm

_____ **10.** You are called to the local high school for a 16-year-old girl who has swallowed an unknown quantity of pills. Which of the following should you inquire about FIRST?
   a. A history of psychiatric care
   b. When the patient took the pills
   c. What kind of pills she took
   d. The patient's estimated weight in kilograms

_____ **11.** A man was trapped in his burning house for approximately 15 minutes before firefighters rescued him. He reports burning in his throat and a severe headache. He has a blood pressure of 180/90 mm Hg, a pulse rate of 120 beats/min, and labored respirations of 28 breaths/min. In addition to providing 100% supplemental oxygen, treatment for this patient should include
   a. amyl nitrate inhaled in 30-second increments.
   b. rapid transport to a local hyperbaric facility.
   c. a slow infusion of sodium nitroprusside.
   d. IV administration of 1 mL/kg of ethyl alcohol.

_____ **12.** You are called to an assisted living facility for a sick resident. The patient, a 70 year-old woman, reports tinnitus and difficulty concentrating. The nurse caring for the resident tells you that she has delivered approximately five cups of ice to the patient's room over the last hour. On the basis of the patient's presentation, you should suspect
a. acute leukemia.
b. chronic anemia.
c. polycythemia.
d. lymphoma.

_____ **13.** When managing a patient with a headache who receives factor VIII therapy, you should be MOST concerned with
a. noting the patient's tendency for chronic hypoxia.
b. obtaining a glucose reading every 15 minutes.
c. avoiding aspirin therapy for the headache.
d. avoiding analgesics of any kind.

_____ **14.** When assessing a patient with abdominal pain, which of the following findings is MOST indicative of peritoneal irritation?
a. Pain that increases when the patient is placed on his or her side
b. A decrease in pain when drawing the knees into the abdomen
c. A relief of pain when the patient moves around frequently
d. Pain that is referred to the shoulder or neck area

_____ **15.** A 60-year-old man reports the sudden onset of excruciating abdominal pain. You provide 100% oxygen via a nonrebreathing mask and prepare the patient for transport. Further management for this patient includes all of the following EXCEPT
a. administering 2 to 4 mg of morphine for pain relief.
b. initiating an IV of normal saline solution.
c. monitoring for signs of shock.
d. assuming that vomiting may occur.

_____ **16.** You are called to a local park where a middle-aged man has collapsed. When you arrive, you find that the patient is disoriented. His skin is hot and moist and his respirations are deep. What is your field impression of this patient?
a. Heat exhaustion
b. Heat prostration
c. Heatstroke
d. Heat cramps

_____ **17.** Which of the following patients would be MOST prone to hypothermia?
a. A 49-year-old man with hyperglycemia
b. A 55-year-old woman with hypothyroidism
c. A 60-year-old woman with hyperthyroidism
d. A 68-year-old man with coronary artery disease

_____ **18.** Care for a patient who reports a severe migraine headache and vomiting includes
   a. transportation in a supine position.
   b. application of heat packs to the head.
   c. administration of prochlorperazine.
   d. IV administration of 10 to 20 mg of morphine sulfate.

_____ **19.** A 55-year-old woman calls EMS because of a "strange feeling." When you arrive, you are met at the door by the patient who appears confused. As your partner is taking her vital signs, she suddenly becomes enraged and yells at you to leave. This patient is MOST likely experiencing a
   a. complex partial seizure.
   b. simple partial seizure.
   c. focal motor seizure.
   d. generalized motor seizure.

_____ **20.** You arrive at the scene of a local community center where a 30-year-old man has been having a seizure for approximately 10 minutes. After the appropriate airway management and the initiation of an IV line, you should administer
   a. 25 g of glucose.
   b. 100 mg of thiamine.
   c. 2 mg of naloxone.
   d. 5 to 10 mg of diazepam.

_____ **21.** Prehospital management for a patient in ventricular fibrillation who has a core body temperature of less than 86°F (30°C) includes
   a. doubling the dose of all cardiac medications.
   b. attempting defibrillation one time at 360 joules.
   c. restricting antiarrhythmic use to lidocaine only.
   d. not intubating until the body temperature rises.

_____ **22.** What is a common finding in both fresh water and salt water drownings?
   a. Pulmonary edema
   b. Loss of surfactant
   c. Inadequate oxygenation
   d. Severe metabolic alkalosis

_____ **23.** Which of the following represents the MOST appropriate field management for a patient with a blood glucose reading of 400 mg/dL and polyuria?
   a. SC administration of 10 units of insulin
   b. Fluid rehydration
   c. 25 g of glucose
   d. IV administration of 40 mg of furosemide

_____ **24.** When assessing a patient who was stung by a bee, which of the following assessment findings would be MOST indicative of anaphylactic shock?
   a. Diaphoretic skin
   b. A fine, red rash
   c. Flushing of the skin
   d. Known allergies to bees

_____ **25.** What is the BEST way to minimize the hypoxia associated with a near drowning?
    a. Immediate intubation
    b. Frequent suctioning of secretions
    c. Prophylactic abdominal thrusts
    d. Rescue breathing while in the water

_____ **26.** A 59-year-old woman with a history of Graves' disease is in a depressed mental state. Her skin is extremely hot to the touch, and she has a pulse rate of 160 beats/min. These findings are MOST consistent with
    a. myxedema.
    b. thyrotoxic crisis.
    c. Addison's disease.
    d. Cushing's syndrome.

_____ **27.** Definitive care for a patient experiencing a "thyroid storm" includes
    a. administrating an adrenergic blockade.
    b. administering glucocorticoids.
    c. initiating fluid resuscitation.
    d. decreasing the blood level of thyroxin.

━━━━━ Questions 28 and 29 pertain to the following scenario:━━━━━

A 23-year-old man was working near a wood pile when he experienced a sudden, sharp pain in his left lower leg. Within 20 minutes, he began experiencing painful spasms of the muscles in his upper legs and abdomen. On EMS arrival, the patient's level of consciousness is markedly diminished.

_____ **28.** The signs and symptoms that this patient is experiencing are MOST likely the result of a bite from a
    a. brown recluse spider.
    b. black widow spider.
    c. rattlesnake or other pit viper.
    d. coral snake.

_____ **29.** In addition to 100% oxygen and possible positive pressure ventilations, management for this patient, based on his symptoms, should include
    a. 10 mL of calcium chloride.
    b. 2.5 to 10 mg of diazepam.
    c. 1 to 2 mg/kg of 10% calcium gluconate.
    d. antivenin derived from goat serum.

_____ **30.** Which of the following conditions would produce the MOST rapid loss of consciousness?
    a. Ketoacidosis
    b. Ischemic stroke
    c. Insulin shock
    d. Hyperglycemia

Subtest 5 Practice Exam: Obstetrics and Pediatrics

_____ **1.** Immediately after delivery, your patient is experiencing heavy vaginal bleeding. To MOST effectively control the bleeding, you should
a. place a trauma dressing inside the vagina.
b. firmly massage the fundus of the uterus.
c. position the mother on her left side.
d. elevate the mother's legs 6"–12".

_____ **2.** You are called by a frantic mother who states that her 2-year-old child is not breathing. When you arrive, you immediately assess for breathing and note that it is absent. After providing two rescue breaths, you should
a. begin chest compressions.
b. prepare to intubate the child.
c. assess for a carotid pulse.
d. assess for a brachial pulse.

_____ **3.** Which of the following parameters is considered LEAST important in the initial assessment of a newborn?
a. Pulse rate
b. Skin color
c. Apgar score
d. Respiratory effort

_____ **4.** A 2-year-old child has fallen from a two-story window. On the basis of the mechanism of injury and the differences in anatomy between a child and an adult, which of the following structures would most likely be injured?
a. Head
b. Chest
c. Abdomen
d. Lower extremities

_____ **5.** When assessing for signs of respiratory distress in an infant, which of the following findings would be MOST indicative of inadequate breathing?
a. Expiratory grunting
b. Abdominal breathing
c. Pulse rate of 120 beats/min
d. Pink oral mucosa

_____ **6.** A 3-year-old child is pulseless and apneic. The ECG shows asystole. What is the MOST appropriate dosage of epinephrine 1:10,000 if given via the IV or IO route?
a. 1 mg/kg
b. 0.1 mg/kg
c. 0.1 mL/kg
d. 0.01 mL/kg

_____ **7.** A woman who is at 38 weeks of gestation has contractions that are 5 minutes apart and lasting approximately 30 seconds each. She tells you that this is her third pregnancy. Which of the following terms describes her obstetric history?
  a. Primigravida
  b. Multipara
  c. Nulligravida
  d. Multigravida

_____ **8.** Which of the following female hormones results in ovulation?
  a. Follicle-stimulating hormone (FSH)
  b. Human chorionic gonadotropin (HCG)
  c. Luteinizing hormone (LH)
  d. Progesterone

_____ **9.** A 26-year-old woman has had abdominal pain since the end of her menstrual period approximately 10 days ago. She reports that the pain is in both lower quadrants, and she has a temperature of 100.5°F (38.0°C). What is the MOST likely cause of her symptoms?
  a. Acute cystitis
  b. Ruptured ovarian cyst
  c. Ectopic pregnancy
  d. Pelvic inflammatory disease

_____ **10.** Management of a woman who has been sexually assaulted should include
  a. cleaning of all nonbleeding wounds.
  b. allowing the patient to take a shower.
  c. recognizing the patient as a crime scene.
  d. allowing a male paramedic to assess the patient.

_____ **11.** A 3-year-old girl has acute respiratory distress following a recent upper respiratory tract infection. Assessment reveals that she is listless and pale, and she has a pulse rate of 70 beats/min. Appropriate initial management should include
  a. IV administration of 0.02 mg/kg of atropine.
  b. use of an aerosolized bronchodilator.
  c. positive pressure ventilations.
  d. 20 mL/kg bolus of normal saline solution.

_____ **12.** You have responded to a call for a 4-year-old girl who has had a seizure. When you arrive, you find that the child is in her mother's arms and crying. Which of the following questions would be the MOST pertinent to ask the mother initially?
  a. Has the child been running a fever?
  b. Does the child have a history of seizures?
  c. Has the child recently had a stiff neck?
  d. Has the child sustained recent head trauma?

_____ **13.** Initial management of a 5-year-old child in status epilepticus should be focused on
  a. administering rectal diazepam.
  b. obtaining a blood glucose reading.
  c. monitoring the pulse rate with electrocardiography.
  d. providing adequate ventilatory support.

_____ **14.** Following delivery, a newborn has a thick dark greenish substance around the mouth. The newborn is crying and has a pulse rate of 120 beats/min. What is the best course of action?
 a. Suction the trachea using an endotracheal tube.
 b. Administer free-flow oxygen and continue your assessment.
 c. Use vigorous stimulation to increase the respiratory rate.
 d. Begin immediate positive pressure ventilations with a BVM device.

_____ **15.** During the delivery of a newborn's head, you note the presence of a nuchal cord. What is the MOST appropriate initial management for this situation?
 a. Gently slip the cord over the newborn's head.
 b. Immediately clamp and cut the cord.
 c. Clamp the cord only and resume with the delivery.
 d. Administer oxygen to the mother and provide rapid transport.

_____ **16.** An 8-year-old male experienced a closed head injury after he fell from the bed of a moving pickup truck. His Glasgow Coma Scale (GCS) score is 7. His respirations are slow and irregular and his pupils are bilaterally dilated and sluggish to react. The MOST appropriate management for this child includes
 a. hyperventilation with a BVM at a rate of 30 breaths/min.
 b. administering 100% oxygen via pediatric nonrebreathing mask.
 c. intubation and ventilations delivered at a rate of 20 breaths/min.
 d. intubation and 2 mg/kg of lidocaine to reduce intracranial pressure.

_____ **17.** You are assessing a 7-year-old boy who has signs of shock. What is the _lower_ limit systolic blood pressure for a child of this age?
 a. 70 to 80 mm Hg
 b. 80 to 85 mm Hg
 c. 85 to 95 mm Hg
 d. 95 to 100 mm Hg

_____ **18.** Which of the following actions would MOST effectively decrease oxygen demand in a small child who is in shock?
 a. Administer epinephrine for hypotension.
 b. Administer 20 mL/kg fluid boluses every 5 minutes.
 c. Take measures to reduce anxiety in the child.
 d. Increase the child's body temperature.

_____ **19.** A patient who is in her third trimester of pregnancy is bleeding. What is the best course of action?
 a. Maintain adequate perfusion.
 b. Provide volume expansion.
 c. Provide positive pressure ventilations.
 d. Massage the fundus of the uterus.

_____ **20.** When performing an assessment on a 3-year-old child, you should be alert to the possibility of abuse if
 a. the child clings to the parent during your assessment.
 b. the child cries during your assessment.
 c. there has been a delay in seeking medical attention for the child.
 d. there are bilateral bruises to the tibial area.

_____ **21.** After providing the appropriate management for a child that you suspect has been physically abused, your next action should be to
  a. notify the police and have the caregiver arrested.
  b. confront the caregiver about your suspicions.
  c. document your suspicions.
  d. report your suspicions to the receiving facility.

_____ **22.** The mother of a 2-year-old girl reports that the child has had a fever for the past 2 days and that she screams every time she tries to pick her up. You note that the child is grabbing both sides of her head. These findings are MOST suggestive of
  a. encephalitis.
  b. meningitis.
  c. dehydration.
  d. impending seizure.

_____ **23.** A 9-year-old child has generalized weakness, blood in the stool, and bruising, even from minor trauma. These findings are MOST consistent with what condition?
  a. Anemia
  b. Lymphoma
  c. Leukemia
  d. Sickle cell disease

_____ **24.** Emergency management for a child with suspected anemia should include
  a. multiple boluses of normal saline solution.
  b. supportive care and transport.
  c. correction of the underlying cause.
  d. immunosuppressant drug therapy.

_____ **25.** What finding is consistent with both HIV infection AND tuberculosis in a child?
  a. Kaposi's sarcoma
  b. *Pneumocystis carinii*
  c. Fever and fatigue
  d. Hemoptysis

_____ **26.** When caring for a child with suspected bacterial meningitis, it is MOST important to
  a. be prepared for seizures.
  b. place a mask on yourself.
  c. monitor the cardiac rhythm.
  d. start an IV at a keep open rate.

You are summoned to a residence for a 7-year-old boy who has had worsening abdominal pain for the past 2 hours. As you enter the house, you find the child lying on the couch with his knees drawn up into his chest. He has a blood pressure of 90/50 mm Hg, a pulse rate of 96 beats/min, and respirations of 28 breaths/min. The child is awake and alert.

_____ **27.** Appropriate assessment of the child's abdomen should include
  a. applying firm pressure to the painful area to determine if peritoneal inflammation is present.
  b. auscultating bowel sounds for approximately 5 minutes to assess for the possibility of a bowel obstruction.
  c. determining the area of pain and focusing on that area, to include palpation, after you have examined the remainder of the abdomen.
  d. palpating the most painful area of the abdomen first so that you can compare it to other less painful areas.

_____ **28.** When transporting the child to the hospital, your priority should be focused on
  a. initiating an IV because of the hypotension.
  b. encouraging the child to remain supine.
  c. administering morphine for pain relief.
  d. getting the child to definitive care.

_____ **29.** As you are assessing the skin color and condition of a newborn, you note that it is red and abnormally warm to the touch. Suspecting fever, you should recall that
  a. postpartum fever in the newborn is a common occurrence.
  b. cooling the child takes priority over all other therapies.
  c. the dose of acetaminophen for a newborn is 15 mg/kg.
  d. this is not a common finding and suggests a significant illness.

_____ **30.** You are caring for a 6-year-old boy with a tracheostomy tube who is in respiratory distress. He has a pulse rate of 70 beats/min, and the pulse oximeter shows a reading of 85%. Immediate care should include
  a. administering epinephrine via the tracheostomy tube.
  b. suctioning the tracheostomy tube.
  c. initiating positive pressure ventilations.
  d. initiating chest compressions.

Subtest 6 Practice Exam: Operations

_____ **1.** While responding to a call for a patient who is in cardiac arrest, you approach an intersection in which you have a red light. What is the MOST appropriate action for the driver to take?
  a. Slow down and proceed cautiously through the red light.
  b. Continue through the red light while looking in both directions.
  c. Stop and wait for the light to turn green prior to proceeding.
  d. Stop to look for oncoming traffic, and then proceed cautiously.

_____ **2.** You and your partner arrive at the scene of a motor vehicle accident, quickly size up the scene, and note that there are two patients, both of which are critically injured. What should you do next?

  a. Immediately load both patients and transport.

  b. Contact medical control and request direction.

  c. Call for a second ambulance to respond to the scene.

  d. Provide management to both patients and transport at once.

_____ **3.** Which of the following scene size-up findings would be MOST indicative of an unsafe environment when approaching a residence?

  a. A dog barking at you as you approach the residence.

  b. The sound of breaking glass coming from the residence.

  c. A very large man who greets you as you approach the residence.

  d. A loud stereo and multiple people making noise inside the residence.

_____ **4.** At the scene of a motor vehicle accident, you note that the driver, a young woman, is lying next to her car and has agonal respirations and no palpable pulse. Other than an open tibial fracture, she has no other obvious trauma. She is wearing a necklace that identifies her as an organ donor. How should you manage this situation?

  a. Begin aggressive management and transport immediately.

  b. Notify the coroner, as the patient is obviously deceased.

  c. Start basic life support and call medical control for advice.

  d. Treat with basic life support and transport her to the hospital.

_____ **5.** Which of the following statements regarding a prehospital care report is true?

  a. The report is not a legal document until it is reviewed by the EMS medical director.

  b. Once a copy of the report is left at the hospital, you cannot write on the front of the form.

  c. A separate addendum is not considered a part of the prehospital care report.

  d. Information in the prehospital care report must include a diagnosis of the patient's condition.

_____ **6.** A middle-aged man reports severe chest pain and is awake and alert to his surroundings. As you are loading him into the ambulance, he tells you that he does not want to go to the hospital. Which of the following statements is MOST correct regarding how to handle this situation?

  a. You advise the patient that once he is in the ambulance, you must transport him to the hospital.

  b. Inform the patient that he can only refuse care if there is a mentally competent witness to assume responsibility for him.

  c. The patient must be transported to the hospital because he is not of sound mind and body.

  d. You must realize that a mentally competent adult can withdraw consent at any time he or she chooses.

_____ **7.** Which of the following situations would MOST likely constitute a case of negligence?
- **a.** A paramedic applies a nasal cannula to a man with respiratory distress who will not tolerate a face mask.
- **b.** A patient involved in a significant motor vehicle accident is not immobilized because he was ambulatory when EMS arrived.
- **c.** A focused physical examination is performed on a patient with an isolated fracture of the left femur.
- **d.** The paramedic must wait 20 minutes at the hospital because a nurse is not available to take a report.

_____ **8.** You are transporting a 34-year-old woman who has severe flank pain that radiates to the groin area. She repeatedly demands that you give her something for the pain. What should you do?
- **a.** Honor the patient's demands and administer a small dose of morphine.
- **b.** Notify medical control and seek guidance on how to manage this situation.
- **c.** Do not give any analgesia because the patient has severe abdominal pain.
- **d.** Give the patient 5 mL of sodium chloride and tell her that it is for the pain.

_____ **9.** Your partner, who is new, is experiencing significant anxiety after a call involving a pediatric cardiac arrest in which the outcome was dubious despite appropriate resuscitative attempts. How can you MOST effectively help your partner?
- **a.** Tell your partner to go home for the rest of the shift and sleep for at least 12 to 18 hours.
- **b.** Send your partner to a busier station so that his or her mind can be taken off the situation.
- **c.** Make sure that your partner understands that most calls end up this way and that he or she must get used to it.
- **d.** Be prepared to spend time with your partner and let him or her talk about the call.

_____ **10.** Which of the following is the MOST effective ways to reduce stress in a patient who is experiencing significant chest pain?
- **a.** Administer diazepam or a similar medication to the patient.
- **b.** Tell the patient that he or she is not having a heart attack.
- **c.** Provide reassurance and a safe comfortable transport.
- **d.** Allow a family member to drive the patient to the hospital.

_____ **11.** A 67-year-old woman who slipped and fell reports pain in her left hip area. Which of the following devices would be MOST effective in moving her?
- **a.** Folding stretcher
- **b.** Stokes basket
- **c.** Ambulance cot
- **d.** Scoop stretcher

_____ **12.** While tending to an unconscious patient who was stabbed in the chest, you notice a knife underneath the patient's left shoulder. Which of the following actions would be MOST appropriate for you to take?
- **a.** Move the knife out of the way so that you can safely tend to the patient.
- **b.** Leave the knife where it is and notify the police as you move the patient.
- **c.** Have a police officer remove the knife as you continue to treat the patient.
- **d.** Pick up the knife and hand it to the police officer that is closest to you.

_____ **13.** You receive a call for a patient who is in cardiac arrest at a nearby residence. When you arrive at the scene, you find an obviously emaciated elderly woman who is pulseless and apneic. As you are preparing to perform your assessment, the patient's husband hands you a questionable piece of paper that states "do not resuscitate." He asks that you take no resuscitative action on his wife. How should manage this situation?
  a. Begin CPR and notify medical control for guidance.
  b. Honor the man's request and do not initiate resuscitation.
  c. Tell the man that you are required to initiate full ACLS measures.
  d. Do not attempt resuscitation until you have notified medical control.

_____ **14.** You receive a call for a young man who has fainted outside of a local restaurant. When you arrive, you see a bystander who has placed a pillow under the patient's head and elevated his legs. The patient is still unconscious. Which of the following questions would be MOST pertinent to ask the bystander?
  a. Are you a certified paramedic?
  b. Is the patient a relative of yours?
  c. Were you a witness to the event?
  d. Does the patient take medications?

_____ **15.** You are transporting a woman with diabetes mellitus who was initially unconscious but improved after the administration of 50% dextrose. The patient is now repeatedly asking you what happened. What should be your MOST appropriate response?
  a. Tell the patient what happened each time she asks.
  b. Advise the patient that you already told her what happened.
  c. Tell the patient that the physician will have to tell her what happened.
  d. Give different information each time to assess the level of consciousness.

_____ **16.** Which of the following examples BEST describes informed consent?
  a. You ask the patient if you have permission to initiate treatment.
  b. You advise the patient of the potential complications of starting an IV.
  c. You initiate treatment with the assumption that the patient would approve.
  d. You inform the patient of the consequences of refusing EMS care.

_____ **17.** You are providing a presentation to a group of non-BLS trained citizens on the importance of calling 9-1-1. What would be the MOST important rationale to explain to the audience for the early notification of EMS?
  a. CPR must be initiated immediately.
  b. Advanced care is the key factor in survival.
  c. The key to increased survival is early defibrillation.
  d. Rapid transport to the hospital saves more lives.

_____ **18.** Important components of a successful public injury prevention program include all of the following EXCEPT
  a. seat belt usage.
  b. rescue breathing.
  c. helmet usage.
  d. pool safety.

_____ **19.** When lifting a patient who is on an ambulance stretcher, you should
  a. position your palms up whenever possible.
  b. keep the muscles of the abdomen relaxed.
  c. avoid using the muscles of your legs.
  d. hold your breath as you lift the patient.

_____ **20.** What is the MOST effective method for preventing the spread of disease?
  a. Always wear gloves with every patient.
  b. Wash your hands frequently, especially in between patients.
  c. Ensure that all of your immunizations are up-to-date.
  d. Wear a mask when caring for patients with tuberculosis.

_____ **21.** When approaching a vehicle in which a patient is slumped over the steering wheel, you should
  a. position the ambulance in front of the vehicle when at all possible.
  b. approach the patient from the front of the car for maximum visibility.
  c. shine a spotlight in the side view mirror until you determine it is safe.
  d. tell the patient to get out of the vehicle so that you may provide care.

_____ **22.** When moving a patient from a house without a carrying device, you should
  a. take long steps to expedite your exit.
  b. walk backwards when moving the patient.
  c. avoid twisting when moving around a corner.
  d. carry the patient over your shoulder if possible.

_____ **23.** Which of the following statements is MOST correct with regards to the proper disposal or handling of sharps?
  a. You should detach the needle from a prefilled syringe prior to disposal.
  b. Dispose of the needle in an appropriate container immediately after use.
  c. Drop the needle on the floor immediately after starting an IV line.
  d. Wait to retrieve and dispose of all sharps until the call is complete.

_____ **24.** What is the ultimate goal of any quality assurance program?
  a. Ensure that high quality care is consistently delivered.
  b. Recognize and reward those personnel with good performance.
  c. Reinforce the strict adherence to all system protocols.
  d. Determine solutions to problems that are identified.

_____ **25.** To ensure the safest response to an emergency scene, you should
  a. use escorts such as a police vehicle whenever it is possible.
  b. have your siren on continuously until you arrive at the scene.
  c. always operate the ambulance with due regard for others.
  d. exceed the speed limit only when responding to a patient who is in cardiac arrest.

_____ **26.** Which of the following would provide the EMT or paramedic with the BEST protection from liability?
  a. Deliver the patient to his or her choice of hospital regardless of the condition.
  b. Maintain a consistently high standard of care when treating all patients.
  c. Treat all patients and their family members with courtesy and respect.
  d. Constantly reinforce your knowledge through continuing education.

_____ **27.** Which of the following situations BEST depicts a case of gross negligence?
   a. When carrying a patient, the paramedic slips and drops the patient.
   b. A paramedic inadvertently intubates a patient's esophagus.
   c. A medication error was made but corrective action was taken.
   d. The defibrillator fails to work because the batteries are dead.

_____ **28.** During a mass-casualty situation, what officer is responsible for communicating with hospitals to ascertain their capabilities?
   a. Staging
   b. Support
   c. Triage
   d. Transport

_____ **29.** Common types of vascular access devices likely to be encountered in a patient receiving home health care include all of the following EXCEPT
   a. central venous devices.
   b. central venous tunneled catheters.
   c. peripherally inserted central catheters.
   d. peripherally inserted IV catheters.

_____ **30.** At the scene of a cardiac arrest, you are unable to contact medical control for authorization to perform a procedure. Which of the following should be your MOST appropriate action?
   a. Continue with basic life support only until you arrive at the hospital.
   b. Follow basic life support procedures until you can make contact.
   c. Follow standard protocols for the procedure that you are requesting.
   d. Elect not to perform the procedure because of the lack of authorization.

Practice Final Examination

_____ **1.** A 30-year-old man who has overdosed on a large quantity of codeine has respirations of 6 breaths/min and a reduction in tidal volume. Which of the following conditions will develop within the first few minutes?
   a. Metabolic alkalosis
   b. Metabolic acidosis
   c. Respiratory acidosis
   d. Respiratory alkalosis

_____ **2.** A 50-year-old man with a self-inflicted gunshot wound to the face has multiple fractures of the mandible, severe oropharyngeal bleeding, and is apneic. Which of the following methods of airway control will be MOST effective for this patient?
   a. Orotracheal intubation
   b. Nasotracheal intubation
   c. Needle cricothyrotomy
   d. BVM device with an oral airway

_____ **3.** An elderly man is unresponsive, and your assessment reveals that he is not breathing. What is the best course of action?
  a. Perform immediate intubation.
  b. Provide two rescue breaths.
  c. Assess his cardiac rhythm.
  d. Assess for a carotid pulse.

_____ **4.** Which of the following medication overdoses could be REVERSED with the administration of naloxone?
  a. Diazepam
  b. Meperidine
  c. Midazolam
  d. Phenobarbitol

_____ **5.** When assessing a patient's pulse, you note that it has an irregularly irregular pattern. On the basis of these findings, which of the following cardiac rhythms would MOST likely be seen on the cardiac monitor?
  a. Sinus tachycardia with a depressed ST segment
  b. Supraventricular tachycardia with aberrant conduction
  c. Second-degree AV block type II with a fixed block
  d. Uncontrolled atrial fibrillation at a rate of 110 to 120 beats/min

━━━━━━━━ **Questions 6–8 pertain to the following scenario:** ━━━━━━━━
A 21-year-old man sustains a large laceration to the left groin area while using a chainsaw. When you arrive, bright red blood is spurting from the wound and the patient is attempting to control the bleeding himself without success.

_____ **6.** After ensuring that the patient's airway is patent and his breathing is adequate, you should
  a. administer 100% oxygen via a nonrebreathing mask.
  b. apply the PASG to control the hemorrhage.
  c. control the bleeding with direct pressure.
  d. apply ice to the wound and elevate the leg.

_____ **7.** Which of the following signs is MOST indicative of early shock?
  a. Rapid, thready pulse
  b. Lethargy or unconsciousness
  c. A drop in systolic blood pressure
  d. Tachypnea with reduced tidal volume

_____ **8.** After the bleeding is controlled, your partner advises you that the patient has a blood pressure of 112/70 mm Hg and a strong pulse rate of 110 beats/min. Which of the following statements regarding IV therapy in this patient is MOST correct?
  a. The patient needs a 2 L bolus of lactated Ringer's solution.
  b. At least one large-bore IV should be started to maintain perfusion.
  c. IV therapy is not indicated because the patient's blood pressure is stable.
  d. Administer 20 mL/kg boluses of normal saline solution until the pulse rate decreases.

_____ **9.** What is the single most important factor in the survivability of sudden cardiac arrest?
   a. Identifying the cause
   b. Effective airway control
   c. Early and effective defibrillation
   d. Immediate transport to the hospital

_____ **10.** After being struck in the head with a baseball bat, a 9-year-old boy immediately loses consciousness. On your arrival, he is conscious but slightly confused. Shortly into your assessment, he lapses into a coma. This scenario and findings are MOST consistent with what type of injury?
   a. Epidural hemorrhage
   b. Subdural hemorrhage
   c. Cerebral contusion
   d. Severe concussion

_____ **11.** When assessing a patient with a closed head injury, you note the presence of trismus. This is defined as
   a. unequal pupils.
   b. unusual breath odor.
   c. clenching of the teeth.
   d. leftward gaze of the eyes.

_____ **12.** A middle-aged man is threatening to kill himself. You see no visible weapons on his person. What should be your initial concern?
   a. Safely transporting him to the hospital
   b. His ability to injure you or your partner
   c. Gathering any medications that he takes
   d. Searching him for a knife or gun

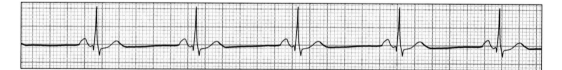

_____ **13.** A 54-year-old man has the above cardiac rhythm. The MOST appropriate initial management should consist of
   a. administering 0.5 mg of atropine sulfate.
   b. preparing for transcutaneous pacing.
   c. determining the patient's hemodynamic status.
   d. starting an IV line at a KVO rate.

_____ **14.** Cardiopulmonary arrest in infants and children is MOST often secondary to
   a. a lethal arrhythmia.
   b. respiratory failure.
   c. severe dehydration.
   d. massive infection.

_____ **15.** You are performing CPR on a 3-month-old infant in asystole. You are unable to initiate an IV but manage to secure an endotracheal tube. Which of the following represents the correct dosage of epinephrine for this infant?
   a. 0.01 mg/kg 1:10,000
   b. 0.01 mL/kg 1:1,000
   c. 0.1 mg/kg 1:1,000
   d. 1.0 mg/kg 1:10,000

_____ **16.** Which of the following findings is MOST suggestive of myxedema?
   a. Hyperthyroidism
   b. Excess thyroxine
   c. Severe hypothermia
   d. Thinning of the skin

_____ **17.** Which of the following BEST describes the sequence of events that precedes cardiac arrest in a drowning episode?
   a. Dysrhythmias, laryngospasm, hypoxia
   b. Laryngospasm, hypoxia, dysrhythmias
   c. Laryngospasm, dysrhythmias, hypoxia
   d. Hypoxia, laryngospasm, dysrhythmias

_____ **18.** A patient who was bitten by a fire ant is unconscious, has severe edema to the face and neck, and generalized urticaria. Breath sounds are difficult to hear, and loud inspiratory stridor is noted. Which of the following management modalities has priority?
   a. Prompt intubation
   b. Administration of epinephrine
   c. Administration of diphenhydramine hydrochloride
   d. Immediate transport

_____ **19.** A 4-year-old child has labored breathing. During your assessment, you note that the pulse rate is 70 beats/min. This pulse rate is
   a. normal for a 4-year-old child.
   b. indicative of increased vagal tone.
   c. significant as it indicates hypoxia.
   d. treated with chest compressions.

_____ **20.** Which of the following statements regarding the use of vasopressin in cardiac arrest is MOST correct?
   a. Vasopressin should be given every 3 to 5 minutes throughout the arrest
   b. Vasopressin is superior to epinephrine and should be used when possible
   c. Vasopressin is highly effective in treating pediatric cardiac arrest patients
   d. Vasopressin can be used to replace the first or second dose of epinephrine

_____ **21.** During resuscitation of a 60-year-old man with pulseless ventricular tachy-cardia, you restore spontaneous circulation following defibrillation, CPR, two doses of epinephrine, and one dose of amiodarone. The patient remains apneic. Which of the following represents the MOST appropriate post-resuscitation care for this patient?
   a. Ventilate at a rate of 10 to 12 breaths/min, obtain a blood pressure, and begin an amiodarone infusion at 1 mg/min
   b. Hyperventilate the patient, administer a 500 mL normal saline bolus, and begin an amiodarone infusion at 0.5 mg/min
   c. Ventilate at a rate of 8 to 10 breaths/min, obtain a blood pressure, and administer 150 mg of amiodarone over 10 minutes
   d. Hyperventilate the patient, begin an epinephrine infusion to maintain perfusion, and administer 1.5 mg/kg of lidocaine

_____ **22.** What is the MOST important concept to explain to a group of non-BLS trained citizens when discussing the importance of rapid EMS notification for a patient in cardiac arrest?
   a. Timely administration of fibrinolytic drugs
   b. Importance of early CPR and defibrillation
   c. Criticality of cardiac medication administration
   d. Rapid EMS transport to an appropriate facility

_____ **23.** You are transporting a patient who has crushing chest pain that is unrelieved by nitroglycerin. You contact medical control for advice and are ordered to administer 25 mg of morphine. Your MOST appropriate response should be to
   a. document the order verbatim and administer the medication.
   b. administer the medication and prepare to intubate the patient.
   c. advise the physician that you believe meperidine hydrochloride would be a better choice.
   d. advise the physician that the dose seems high and request clarification.

_____ **24.** Assessment and management of a conscious woman with suspected cardiac-related chest pain might include all of the following EXCEPT
   a. obtaining a 12-lead electrocardiogram.
   b. asking the patient if she has a cardiac history.
   c. performing a quick look with the defibrillator.
   d. inquiring as to when the patient last ate.

_____ **25.** A 40-year-old construction worker fell approximately 10′ and sustained an open fracture of the left femur. Further examination reveals that the distal femur is protruding through the skin. What is the MOST appropriate care for this injury?
   a. Cover the wound with a sterile dressing and immobilize the leg.
   b. Apply a traction splint and cover the wound.
   c. Provide manual traction until the fracture is reduced.
   d. Immobilize the leg in a flexed position and provide transport.

_____ **26.** What is the MOST appropriate device to use on a patient with respiratory difficulty who has a reduction in tidal volume?
   a. Nasal cannula at 1 to 6 L/min
   b. Nonrebreathing mask at 15 L/min
   c. BVM device with supplemental oxygen
   d. Oxygen powered transport ventilator

_____ **27.** Which of the following assessment findings would indicate the MOST patent airway?
   a. Diaphoresis and a forceful cough
   b. Gurgling respirations and cyanosis
   c. Semiconscious with snoring respirations
   d. Loud inspiratory stridor and severe pallor

———— **Questions 28–30 pertain to the following scenario:** ————

You are dispatched to a local ranch where a tractor has overturned and pinned the operator. While en route, a law enforcement officer at the scene advises you that a 60-year-old man is trapped at the legs by the tractor. On the basis of this information, you request the fire department for heavy rescue.

_____ **28.** On arrival at the scene, your FIRST priority should be to
   a. direct your partner to stabilize the patient's head.
   b. determine whether or not there are any dangers.
   c. assess the degree to which the patient is entrapped.
   d. assess the patient's breathing and provide oxygen.

_____ **29.** Once at the patient's side, you note that his level of consciousness is markedly decreased. What should you do next?
   a. Apply 100% oxygen with a nonrebreathing mask.
   b. Initiate two large-bore IVs with normal saline solution.
   c. Perform a jaw-thrust maneuver to ensure a patent airway.
   d. Begin some form of positive pressure ventilations.

_____ **30.** You note that the patient's respiratory rate is 20 breaths/min and eupneic. What is the MOST appropriate next step?
   a. Continue with your assessment.
   b. Apply 100% supplemental oxygen.
   c. Initiate ventilatory assistance.
   d. Auscultate the patient's lungs.

Questions 31-33 pertain to the following scenario:

After determining that an elderly man is pulseless and apneic, you assess the cardiac rhythm and note the following:

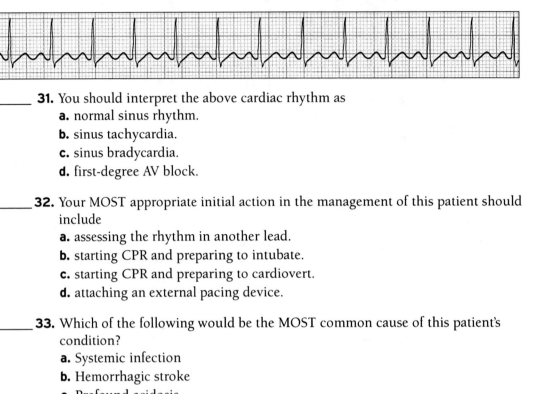

_____ **31.** You should interpret the above cardiac rhythm as
    a. normal sinus rhythm.
    b. sinus tachycardia.
    c. sinus bradycardia.
    d. first-degree AV block.

_____ **32.** Your MOST appropriate initial action in the management of this patient should include
    a. assessing the rhythm in another lead.
    b. starting CPR and preparing to intubate.
    c. starting CPR and preparing to cardiovert.
    d. attaching an external pacing device.

_____ **33.** Which of the following would be the MOST common cause of this patient's condition?
    a. Systemic infection
    b. Hemorrhagic stroke
    c. Profound acidosis
    d. Severe hypercalcemia

_____ **34.** A patient with diabetic ketoacidosis would typically present with which of the following signs and/or symptoms?
    a. Hypoglycemia and dehydration
    b. Hypoglycemia and polyuria
    c. Hyperglycemia and dehydration
    d. Hyperglycemia and oliguria

_____ **35.** What is your FIRST priority in caring for a patient with a swollen, painful, and deformed left forearm?
    a. Immobilize the injury.
    b. Prevent further injury.
    c. Assess distal pulses.
    d. Align the deformity.

_____ **36.** You are aggressively managing a patient who sustained severe trauma to the chest following a head-on collision with a tree. Assessment reveals an initial blood pressure of 100/60 mm Hg, a pulse rate of 120 beats/min, and respirations of 28 breaths/min. Which of the following repeat vital signs would be MOST suggestive of a pericardial tamponade?
    a. BP of 80/40, pulse rate of 120
    b. BP of 90/70, pulse rate of 128
    c. BP of 104/70, pulse rate of 100
    d. BP of 160/90, pulse rate of 90

_____ **37.** You are assisting in the delivery of a baby. As soon as the head delivers, you should
  a. suction the oropharynx and then the nose.
  b. apply gentle pressure to the top of the head.
  c. guide the head up to deliver the lower shoulder.
  d. briskly dry the baby's face off to stimulate breathing.

_____ **38.** You are called to care for a 3-year-old child with a fever who has had a seizure. Management should consist of
  a. rapid cooling in cool water.
  b. administration of 0.5 mg/kg diazepam rectally.
  c. initiating an IV of normal saline solution.
  d. supportive care and transport.

_____ **39.** Which of the following findings is considered a reliable early indicator of shock in a 2-year-old child?
  a. Confusion and anxiety
  b. Delayed capillary refill
  c. Slow, bounding pulse rate
  d. Rapid, weak pulse rate

_____ **40.** Which of the following is considered appropriate body substance isolation precautions when caring for an AIDS patient with abdominal pain?
  a. Gloves only
  b. Gloves and a mask
  c. Gloves, gown, and a mask
  d. Gloves and a HEPA mask

_____ **41.** As you are managing an elderly woman who is in cardiac arrest, a man approaches you and states that the patient is his mother and that she did not want to be resuscitated. What is the MOST appropriate course of action?
  a. Ask for a DNR order and if produced, cease your efforts.
  b. Transport the patient to the hospital, providing BLS only.
  c. Politely ask the man to leave and resume resuscitation.
  d. Continue resuscitation and ask for a valid living will.

_____ **42.** Angioneurotic edema is a common finding in a patient who is having a severe allergic reaction. This can pose an immediate threat to life secondary to
  a. compartment syndrome.
  b. congestive heart failure.
  c. intracranial pressure.
  d. airway compromise.

_____ **43.** A 49-year-old man has a headache and reports that he has had visual disturbances that have progressively worsened over the past 2 months. These symptoms are MOST consistent with which of the following conditions?
  a. Subdural hemorrhage
  b. Cerebral neoplasm
  c. Epidural hematoma
  d. Bacterial meningitis

_____ **44.** After delivering a baby, you clear the airway and provide measures to prevent hypothermia. As you assess the newborn, you note the presence of central cyanosis and a pulse rate of 90 beats/min. Immediate management for this newborn should include
a. chest compressions.
b. tactile stimulation.
c. positive pressure ventilations.
d. intubation and tracheal suctioning.

———— Questions 45-48 pertain to the following scenario: ————
You are called to a private residence for a 60-year-old woman who reports respiratory difficulty. On arrival, the clearly anxious woman tells you that she was suddenly awakened with the feeling that she was being smothered. You can see traces of dried blood on her lips.

_____ **45.** After calming the patient, you convince her to sit in a chair as you begin your assessment. She has slight perioral cyanosis and a rapid pulse rate. The pulse oximeter reads 90%. Your initial action should be to
a. attach a cardiac monitor.
b. auscultate breath sounds.
c. apply supplemental oxygen.
d. administer a bronchodilator.

The patient is displaying the cardiac rhythm shown below. She has a blood pressure of 88/60 mm Hg, and she is still in significant respiratory distress.

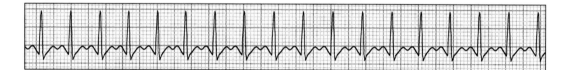

_____ **46.** You should interpret the above cardiac rhythm as
a. supraventricular tachycardia.
b. uncontrolled atrial fibrillation.
c. atrial flutter with a fixed block.
d. ventricular tachycardia.

_____ **47.** What is the MOST appropriate management for this rhythm?
a. Defibrillation with 200 joules
b. Prompt transcutaneous pacing
c. 150 mg of amiodarone
d. Sedation and cardioversion

_____ **48.** Which of the following pathophysiologies BEST explains this woman's respiratory distress?
a. Increased stroke volume with right heart failure
b. Increased preload with left heart failure
c. Decreased preload with right heart failure
d. Decreased stroke volume with left heart failure

Questions 49 and 50 relate to the same patient.

_____ **49.** A 56-year-old man has had chest pain for the past 2 days. His wife calls EMS when she notices that he is not acting right. Your assessment reveals that he has a blood pressure of 80/40 mm Hg, his skin is diaphoretic, and his pulse is weak and rapid. These findings are MOST consistent with which of the following conditions?
   a. Acute ischemic stroke
   b. Unstable angina pectoris
   c. Cardiogenic hypoperfusion
   d. Acute myocardial infarction

_____ **50.** After providing the appropriate airway management, securing an IV line, and administering a brief trial of fluids in an attempt to raise the blood pressure, you should administer which of the following medications?
   a. 2 to 20 µg/kg/min of dopamine
   b. 2 to 10 µg/min of epinephrine
   c. 150 mg of amiodarone in 50 mL D5W
   d. 2 µg/min infusion of nitroglycerin

_____ **51.** Which of the following airway interventions is NOT appropriate for use in children?
   a. Endotracheal intubation
   b. Laryngeal mask airway
   c. Pharyngeal tracheal lumen airway
   d. Surgical or needle cricothyrotomy

_____ **52.** When assessing a deeply unconscious patient, you note the absence of breathing. What method of airway management is contraindicated?
   a. Blind nasotracheal intubation
   b. Esophageal Combitube
   c. Endotracheal intubation
   d. Laryngeal mask airway

_____ **53.** What is the MOST effective way to reduce the morbidity and mortality resulting from trauma?
   a. Limit on scene time to no more than 10 minutes.
   b. Recognize and manage the early signs of shock.
   c. Immediately transport patients with a significant MOI.
   d. Coordinate and conduct injury prevention programs.

_____ **54.** When an adult is struck by an automobile, a typical sequence of events includes the person turning
   a. away from the vehicle and being propelled away from the car.
   b. away from the vehicle and being thrown onto the hood.
   c. towards the vehicle and being thrown onto the hood.
   d. towards the vehicle and being propelled away from the car.

_____ **55.** The initial trauma sustained by a person because of an explosion is usually the result of
   a. flying projectiles.
   b. the pressure wave.
   c. being thrown into structures.
   d. widespread burns to the body.

_____ **56.** Patients with which of the following disease processes represent the highest population that receive home health care?
  a. Malignancies
  b. Infectious diseases
  c. Diabetes mellitus
  d. Psychiatric disorders

_____ **57.** What disease primarily affects low birth weight infants and is characterized by ongoing respiratory distress, frequent lower respiratory tract infections, and the requirement for mechanical ventilation?
  a. Cystic fibrosis
  b. Myasthenia gravis
  c. Congestive heart failure
  d. Bronchopulmonary dysplasia

_____ **58.** Which of the following statements would be inappropriate to document on a patient care form?
  a. "The patient stated that he is HIV positive."
  b. "The patient appears to need psychiatric help."
  c. "The possible smell of ETOH was noted at the scene."
  d. "The patient became very combative on assessment."

_____ **59.** A 16-year-old girl was bitten by a rattlesnake on the lateral aspect of her left lower leg while hiking. She is conscious but reports weakness. She has a blood pressure of 92/56 mm Hg and a pulse rate of 120 beats/min. Management should consist of
  a. placing the patient in a semisitting position.
  b. positioning the extremity above the level of the heart.
  c. initiating an IV of normal saline solution and providing prompt transport.
  d. applying ice to the bite area and immobilizing the entire extremity.

_____ **60.** Which of the following patients is at HIGHEST risk for suicide?
  a. A man who owns multiple guns and knives
  b. A man who has not slept for 72 hours
  c. A woman whose mother committed suicide
  d. A woman who is undergoing a divorce

_____ **61.** Your priority in managing a patient with a behavioral or psychiatric crisis includes
  a. ensuring personal safety and taking BSI precautions.
  b. avoiding any confrontation with the patient.
  c. providing safe transportation to the hospital.
  d. managing any concomitant medical problems.

_____ **62.** At the scene of a violent crime, a patient has been decapitated with an axe. Which of the following is considered the MOST appropriate way for you to manage this situation?
  a. Apply a cardiac monitor to verify asystole.
  b. Do not touch the body if at all possible.
  c. Assess the body for other injuries.
  d. Contact the patient's family.

_____ **63.** Which of the following generally is NOT a role or responsibility of the EMS medical director?
  a. Responding to the scene with the EMTs or paramedics
  b. Defining the scope of practice for EMTs and paramedics
  c. Participating actively in the quality assurance program
  d. Ensuring that all personnel are trained and educated

_____ **64.** An off-duty paramedic stops at the scene of a cardiac arrest on the highway. During the course of providing care to the patient, the paramedic performs endotracheal intubation. Which of the following statements is MOST correct regarding the paramedic's actions?
  a. The paramedic performed in accordance with the standard of care for his level of training.
  b. Since the paramedic was off duty, he is protected by the Good Samaritan laws.
  c. The paramedic could be held liable for practicing medicine without a license.
  d. The paramedic will be legally covered provided that he notifies the medical director after the occurrence.

_____ **65.** You are summoned to the residence of an 18-year-old man with respiratory distress. On arrival, the patient's mother greets you and states that her son recently had a "falling out" with his girlfriend. You assess the patient, who is awake and alert, and note the presence of carpopedal spasms to his hands and a respiratory rate of 40 breaths/min. Initial management for this patient should consist of
  a. applying 100% oxygen with a nonrebreathing mask.
  b. providing coaching to slow the patient's breathing.
  c. administering a sedative drug to help calm the patient.
  d. applying an oxygen mask with the flow rate set at 2 L/min.

_____ **66.** A 49-year-old man has acute shortness of breath. He is awake but is gasping for air. A pulse oximeter reads 84% on room air. Initial management should consist of
  a. some form of ventilatory assistance.
  b. 100% oxygen with a nonrebreathing mask.
  c. sedation and endotracheal intubation.
  d. maintenance of airway patency with an oral airway.

_____ **67.** Assessment of a patient with acute respiratory distress reveals that he is alert but wheezing on exhalation. In addition to oxygen, management should include
  a. intubation before the airway swells.
  b. administration of 3 to 5 mg of epinephrine subcutaneously.
  c. administration of an inhaled beta-agonist medication.
  d. administration of a beta-blocker, such as metoprolol tartrate.

_____ **68.** Management of a patient with an acute asthma attack should focus on which of the following goals?
  a. Rehydration and oxygenation
  b. Determination and correction of the cause
  c. Prompt transport to the nearest hospital
  d. Relief of the bronchospasm and improved ventilation

_____ **69.** Which of the following signs or symptoms would you expect to see in a patient with acetylcholinesterase inhibition secondary to poisoning?
   a. Extreme hyperactivity
   b. Acute urinary retention
   c. Excessive salivation
   d. Pupillary dilation

_____ **70.** A 34-year-old woman has overdosed on a combination of amitriptyline hydrochloride and diazepam, and she has shallow respirations of 8 breaths/min. What is the MOST appropriate management?
   a. Naloxone and sodium bicarbonate
   b. Naloxone, flumazenil, and ventilatory assistance
   c. Sodium bicarbonate and flumazenil
   d. Sodium bicarbonate and ventilatory assistance

_____ **71.** An unconscious trauma patient has snoring respirations. You can see visible blood bubbling from the patient's mouth. What should be your FIRST action?
   a. Suction the oropharynx
   b. Perform a jaw-thrust maneuver
   c. Assist ventilations
   d. Roll the patient to the side

_____ **72.** A 39-year-old man, who weighs approximately 160 pounds, was trapped inside his burning house and sustained full-thickness burns to approximately 40% of his body. On the basis of the Parkland formula, how much IV crystalloid solution should he receive within the first hour?
   a. 620 mL
   b. 700 mL
   c. 730 mL
   d. 815 mL

_____ **73.** An important aspect in the management of a patient with extensive full-thickness burns includes
   a. cooling the burned areas with saline solution.
   b. taking steps to prevent hyperthermia.
   c. performing continuous assessment of the airway.
   d. performing a needle cricothyrotomy.

_____ **74.** Which of the following is considered an effective method in reducing stress in an obviously anxious bystander at the scene of an emergency?
   a. Assign the bystander minor, nonpatient care-related tasks.
   b. Advise the bystander to keep at a safe distance and observe.
   c. Use the bystander for tasks such as crowd and traffic control.
   d. Tell the bystander that he or she should leave the scene at once.

_____ **75.** You are providing care to a patient with suspected cardiac chest pain and elect to start an IV line; however, you did not advise the patient of this ahead of time. As a result, you could be held liable for
   a. assault.
   b. battery.
   c. breach of duty.
   d. proximate cause.

_____ **76.** A 65-year-old man has crushing chest pain that is unrelieved after taking three nitroglycerin tablets. The patient is awake and alert to his surroundings. You assess his vital signs and find him to be significantly hypertensive. As your partner is preparing the stretcher, the patient tells you that he does not want to go to the hospital. After multiple attempts to convince the patient to allow you to transport him, he still refuses. Which of the following represents the MOST appropriate way to manage this situation?
   a. Advise the patient that he should follow-up with his doctor.
   b. Tell the patient that his refusal could ultimately result in death.
   c. Advise the patient that he is too scared to make such a decision.
   d. Refer him to a local after hour's clinic to have an ECG performed.

_____ **77.** In performing a rapid trauma assessment on a young man who fell approximately 25′, you should assess the chest for
   a. distention and rigidity.
   b. crepitus and distention.
   c. symmetry and tenderness.
   d. lung sounds and distention.

_____ **78.** You arrive at the scene approximately 8 minutes after a 51-year-old male collapsed at a family event. Family members are gathered around the patient; however, nobody has provided any care prior to your arrival. After determining that the patient is pulseless and apneic, you should
   a. perform a precordial thump and then assess his cardiac rhythm.
   b. begin CPR and immediately load the patient into the ambulance.
   c. assess his cardiac rhythm after performing about 2 minutes of CPR.
   d. defibrillate the patient immediately and then assess for a carotid pulse.

_____ **79.** When managing a patient in ventricular fibrillation, you elect to administer amiodarone. Which of the following represents the correct dosage and rate of administration for this medication?
   a. 150 mg in 50 mL D5W given over 20 minutes
   b. 150 mg in 100 mL D5W given over 10 minutes
   c. 300 mg administered over 2 to 3 minutes
   d. 300 mg via rapid IV push

_____ **80.** A trauma patient has signs of hypoperfusion but exhibits no external signs of injury. You should suspect which of the following injuries?
   a. Bleeding into the pelvic cavity
   b. Intrathoracic hemorrhage
   c. Retroperitoneal hemorrhage
   d. Intracerebral hemorrhage

_____ **81.** The pneumatic antishock garment (PASG) is clearly indicated in which of the following situations?
   a. Pelvic instability with significant hypotension
   b. Bilateral femur fractures in a patient with congestive heart failure
   c. Blunt chest trauma with signs of hypoperfusion
   d. Open abdominal trauma with severe bleeding

_____82. When assessing a patient with suspected cardiac-related chest pain, which of the following questions would be MOST appropriate to ask?
a. Does the pain move to your arms?
b. Is this the worst pain of your life?
c. Is the pain crushing or dull in nature?
d. Can you describe the quality of the pain?

_____83. Which of the following medication regimens represents the MOST correct sequence when managing a patient with a suspected acute myocardial infarction?
a. Oxygen, nitroglycerin, aspirin, and morphine
b. Oxygen, morphine, aspirin, and nitroglycerin
c. Oxygen, aspirin, nitroglycerin, and morphine
d. Oxygen, aspirin, morphine, and nitroglycerin

_____84. You are preparing to defibrillate a patient in cardiac arrest with a manual biphasic defibrillator, but are unsure of the appropriate initial energy setting. What should you do?
a. Contact medical control for further guidance.
b. Deliver three sequential shocks with 120 joules.
c. Deliver one shock with 200 joules and resume CPR.
d. Continue CPR and shock with 360 joules in 2 minutes.

_____85. What is the MOST appropriate action to take when you suspect child abuse?
a. Provide thorough objective documentation.
b. Report your suspicions to the police.
c. Apprise the parents of your suspicions.
d. Transport the child against the parent's wishes.

_____86. You are managing a violent patient when it is determined that restraints are necessary. When applying the restraints, you should be MOST concerned with
a. preventing positional asphyxia.
b. restraining the patient in a prone position.
c. ensuring that there are at least two people to assist.
d. talking to the patient during the process.

_____87. Assessment of a 6-month-old infant reveals lethargy, absence of tearing, and dry mucous membranes. Which of the following represents the MOST appropriate rate for fluid rehydration?
a. 10 mL/kg
b. 20 mL/kg
c. 125 mL/h
d. 200-mL bolus

──────── **Questions 88-91 pertain to the following scenario:**────────
You are called to a local supermarket where a customer collapsed while paying for his groceries. The man is approximately 50 years of age and appears to weigh about 180 lb. When you arrive, two bystanders are performing CPR.

_____**88.** Once at the patient's side, your FIRST action should be to
    a. verify the effectiveness of the bystander's CPR.
    b. immediately perform a quick look with the defibrillator.
    c. assess the patient to confirm the presence of cardiac arrest.
    d. perform a precordial thump and assess for a carotid pulse.

The ECG reveals the following cardiac rhythm:

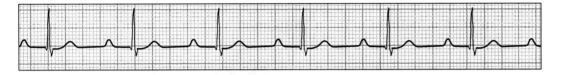

_____**89.** Noting the above rhythm, your next MOST appropriate action should be to
    a. tell the bystanders to continue CPR.
    b. prepare to initiate external pacing.
    c. continue CPR and initiate an IV line.
    d. assess for the presence of a pulse.

_____**90.** Which of the following represents the MOST appropriate initial drug and dose that is given to all adult patients in cardiac arrest?
    a. 40 units of vasopressin every 3 to 5 minutes
    b. 0.1 mg/kg of epinephrine every 3 to 5 minutes
    c. 1 mg of epinephrine 1:10,000 every 3 to 5 minutes
    d. 10 mL of epinephrine 1:1,000 every 3 to 5 minutes

_____**91.** Immediately following placement of an endotracheal tube in this patient, what is the FIRST action that you should take?
    a. Begin ventilating and auscultate breath sounds.
    b. Attach an end-tidal carbon dioxide detector.
    c. Instill 0.1 mL/kg of epinephrine down the ET tube.
    d. Inflate the distal cuff of the tube with 5 to 10 mL of air.

_____**92.** What are the therapeutic effects of morphine sulfate when administered to a patient with cardiogenic pulmonary edema?
    a. Increased venous capacitance and decreased preload
    b. Increased cardiac inotropy and increased cardiac output
    c. Decreased venous capacitance and increased inotropy
    d. Systemic venous pooling of blood and increased afterload

_____**93.** Which of the following findings would be MOST suggestive of right-sided heart failure?
    a. Persistent orthopnea
    b. Blood-tinged sputum
    c. Nocturnal dyspnea
    d. Engorged jugular veins

_____ **94.** During your SAMPLE history of an elderly man, he tells you that his cardiologist told him that he has an "irregular heartbeat." His medications include warfarin sodium and digoxin. On the basis of this information, what underlying cardiac rhythm should you suspect?
   a. Atrial flutter
   b. Atrial fibrillation
   c. Atrial tachycardia
   d. Wandering atrial pacemaker

———— Questions 95–100 pertain to the following scenario:————

A middle-aged man walks into your EMS station reporting heaviness about his chest, shortness of breath, and palpitations. You sit him down and begin to assess him. As your partner is applying 100% supplemental oxygen, the patient tells you that he underwent triple bypass surgery approximately 3 years ago but has been doing fine until now. His blood pressure is 116/58 mm Hg and his pulse is rapid and weak.

_____ **95.** As your partner is attaching the ECG leads, your next action should be to
   a. initiate an IV line.
   b. administer 2 to 4 mg of morphine IM.
   c. administer up to 325 mg of aspirin.
   d. administer 0.4 mg of nitroglycerin.

_____ **96.** The patient tells you that he takes enalapril maleate. What type of medication is this?
   a. ACE inhibitor
   b. Beta-blocker
   c. Calcium channel blocker
   d. Parasympathetic blocker

After placing the patient on a cardiac monitor, you note the following rhythm:

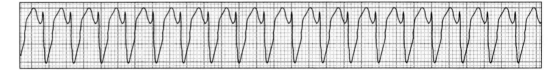

_____ **97.** After noting the above cardiac rhythm, you immediately reassess the patient. He is confused, diaphoretic, and has a blood pressure of 80/50 mm Hg. A patent IV line is in place. What is your next MOST appropriate action?
   a. Administer 150 mg of amiodarone over 10 minutes
   b. Attempt vagal maneuvers and then consider adenosine
   c. Consider sedation and then cardiovert with 100 joules
   d. Administer a 500-mL normal saline bolus and reassess

_____ **98.** As you are administering the therapy in question #97, the patient suddenly loses consciousness. What should you do FIRST?
   a. Perform a head tilt-chin lift maneuver.
   b. Assess for a carotid pulse.
   c. Assess the patient's breathing.
   d. Deliver a precordial thump.

_____ **99.** You note that the patient has agonal respirations. What is the MOST appropriate management at this point?
   a. Apply a face mask with 100% oxygen.
   b. Begin rescue breathing with a pocket mask.
   c. Perform immediate endotracheal intubation.
   d. Visualize the airway for any obstructions.

The patient is pulseless and the monitor displays the following rhythm:

_____**100.** The MOST appropriate initial management for the above rhythm should include
   a. synchronized cardioversion.
   b. defibrillation at 360 joules.
   c. CPR for 30 to 60 seconds.
   d. IV administration of 1 to 1.5 mg of lidocaine.

_____ **101.** When transporting a patient for a prolonged period of time on a nasal cannula, you should
   a. set the flow rate to at least 4 L/min.
   b. vary the liter flow from 1 to 6 L/min.
   c. attach an oxygen humidifier.
   d. ensure that the patient is supine.

_____**102.** A patient in cardiac arrest arrives at the emergency department via EMS. Initial arterial blood gas analysis shows a pH of 7.1, a PO_2 of 90 mm Hg, and a PCO_2 of 58 mm Hg. These findings are MOST consistent with
   a. metabolic acidosis.
   b. metabolic alkalosis.
   c. respiratory alkalosis.
   d. respiratory acidosis.

_____**103.** On the basis of the blood gas readings in question #102, you should expect which of the following management modalities to occur next?
   a. Sodium bicarbonate at 1 mEq/kg
   b. Increased tidal volume and increased breath rate
   c. Decreased tidal volume and increased breath rate
   d. An overall decrease in ventilatory rate

_____**104.** A 17-year-old girl is ejected from the car during a high-speed motor vehicle accident. You find her in a supine position lying motionless, conscious, and confused. She has a blood pressure of 80/40 mm Hg, a pulse rate of 58 beats/min, and respirations of 28 breaths/min. You should treat this patient for
   a. neurogenic shock.
   b. hypovolemic shock.
   c. severe head injury.
   d. unstable bradycardia.

_____ **105.** The diaphoresis seen in patients with shock is the result of
   a. peripheral vasoconstriction.
   b. shunting of blood from the skin.
   c. increased secretion by the sweat glands.
   d. decreased peripheral vascular resistance.

_____ **106.** What is the MOST common reason why victims of spousal abuse do not report the crime?
   a. Inconvenience
   b. Fear of repercussion
   c. Love for the spouse
   d. Feelings of guilt

_____ **107.** While assessing an elderly woman who fell, you note crepitus and pain to the pelvis. No other injuries are noted. The patient is conscious but very restless, and her skin is dry. You take her vital signs and note that she is dangerously hypotensive with a pulse rate of 60 beats/min. Which of the following would BEST explain her vital sign findings?
   a. The elderly generally do not respond to shock with tachycardia.
   b. She takes a beta-blocker for hypertension and atrial fibrillation.
   c. The patient has most likely sustained head trauma as well.
   d. She has sustained spinal injury and is in neurogenic shock.

_____ **108.** While intubating a 44-year-old man in respiratory failure, you note that his pulse rate increases during the procedure. What should be your next MOST appropriate action?
   a. Discontinue the intubation attempt and hyperventilate the patient for 2 to 3 minutes.
   b. Continue with intubation as your partner performs a carotid sinus massage.
   c. Recognize this as a normal response during intubation and monitor the pulse rate.
   d. Complete the intubation attempt and administer adenosine after the tube is secured.

_____ **109.** A 66-year-old woman is diagnosed with cardiomyopathy. What does this indicate?
   a. An enlarged myocardium
   b. Progressive cardiac weakening
   c. Strengthening of the ventricles
   d. An occluded coronary artery

_____ **110.** Possible side effects of the administration of atropine sulfate include
   a. hypotension.
   b. hypersalivation.
   c. pupillary constriction.
   d. acute urinary retention.

_____ **111.** A selective beta$_2$-adrenergic agonist will produce which of the following effects?
   a. Bronchodilation
   b. Increased inotropy
   c. Increased vascular resistance
   d. A parasympathetic effect on the heart

_____ **112.** When treating a narrow complex tachycardia in an adult, the total cumulative dose of adenosine should not exceed
   a. 12 mg.
   b. 18 mg.
   c. 30 mg.
   d. 36 mg.

_____ **113.** When administering a sympathomimetic medication, you should be MOST alert for
   a. severe bradycardia.
   b. cardiac arrhythmias.
   c. acute hypotension.
   d. acute respiratory failure.

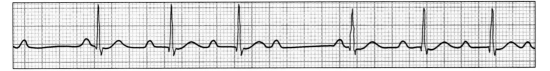

_____ **114.** You should interpret the above cardiac rhythm as
   a. wandering atrial pacemaker.
   b. complete AV dissociation.
   c. type I second-degree AV block.
   d. type II second-degree AV block.

_____ **115.** Low-grade fever and respiratory distress with a slow onset in a 1-year-old infant is MOST characteristic of
   a. croup.
   b. asthma.
   c. epiglottitis.
   d. bronchitis.

_____ **116.** You are assessing a semiconscious man's respirations and note that he is taking irregular breaths that vary in volume and rate with periods of apnea. This breathing pattern is MOST consistent with
   a. Biot's respirations.
   b. agonal respirations.
   c. Kussmaul's respirations.
   d. Cheyne-Stokes respirations.

_____ **117.** In which of the following traumatic injuries would you be MOST likely to encounter pulsus paradoxus?
   a. Tension pneumothorax
   b. Pericardial tamponade
   c. Massive hemothorax
   d. Traumatic asphyxia

_____ **118.** A 39-year-old man is pulseless and apneic after having been lost in the woods for 3 days during the middle of winter. He has a core body temperature of 80°F (26.6°C). In managing this patient, you should avoid
a. defibrillation.
b. intubation.
c. chest compressions.
d. cardiac medications.

_____ **119.** You are summoned to a residence for a patient who has difficulty breathing. At the scene, you are greeted by a young man who escorts you to the bedroom where you find an emaciated 30-year-old man lying in bed. He is diaphoretic and states that he has been running a fever for the past 10 days. You note the appearance of purplish blotches on his arms and neck. Which of the following disease processes should you be MOST highly suspicious of?
a. Tuberculosis
b. Pneumonia
c. HIV/AIDS
d. Hepatitis

_____ **120.** A 60-year-old man reports dyspnea. While auscultating his chest, you hear fine, moist, thin sounds in all lung fields. What is this MOST suggestive of?
a. Fluid in the small lower airways
b. Fluid in the large lower airways
c. Mucous plugs in the alveoli
d. Mild to moderate bronchospasm

_____ **121.** Which of the following patients could you legally treat and transport without consent?
a. An adult patient who is now alert after the administration of dextrose
b. A 16-year-old married girl who is awake and alert after falling
c. A 17-year-old conscious boy who sustained a fractured femur
d. A 6-month-old infant in respiratory distress whose parents refuse care

_____ **122.** A 30-year-old man has sustained multisystem trauma after being struck by a car that was traveling at a high rate of speed. Which of the following elements of care is MOST critical to his survival?
a. Providing high concentrations of oxygen
b. Limiting on-scene time and providing rapid transport
c. Starting at least one large-bore IV line
d. Being in constant contact with medical control

_____ **123.** A 40-year-old woman who was recently discharged from the hospital reports the sudden onset of difficulty breathing and sharp chest pain that increases with breathing. Her skin is cyanotic and diaphoretic, and the pulse oximeter reads 82%. What is the most likely diagnosis?
a. Spontaneous pneumothorax
b. Acute bacterial pneumonia
c. Acute pulmonary embolism
d. Acute pulmonary artery rupture

_____**124.** When assessing a patient's pulse, you should note which of the following?
   a. Rate, strength, and equality
   b. Rate, regularity, and quality
   c. Rate, rhythm, and strength
   d. Rate, regularity, and equality

_____**125.** What is your ultimate goal in caring for a patient with an acute psychiatric crisis?
   a. Obtain as much information as you can.
   b. Determine if the patient is a threat to himself or herself.
   c. Safely transport the patient to the hospital.
   d. Gather all medications that the patient is taking.

_____**126.** A function of the hypothalamus includes
   a. controlling appetite.
   b. influencing respirations.
   c. influencing emotions and level of awareness.
   d. maintaining equilibrium and balance.

_____**127.** While transporting a 50-year-old man in severe respiratory distress, he suddenly gets off of the stretcher, stands up, and pulls the oxygen mask from his face. How should you MOST appropriately manage this situation?
   a. Place the patient supine and assist ventilations.
   b. Administer 5 to 10 mg of diazepam to calm the patient.
   c. Apply a nasal cannula and try to calm the patient.
   d. Perform a rapid sequence induction and intubation.

──────── **Questions 128–132 pertain to the following scenario:** ────────

You and your partner receive a call for a woman in labor. The closest hospital from the patient's residence is approximately 25 miles away. When you arrive at the scene, the anxious husband meets you at the door and tells you that he thinks the baby will deliver at any time.

_____**128.** After making contact with the patient, you determine that she is gravida-4 and para-3. On the basis of this information, how many children does she have?
   a. 2
   b. 3
   c. 4
   d. 6

_____**129.** To determine whether or not delivery is imminent, which of the following questions would be MOST pertinent for you to ask the mother?
   a. Has your amniotic sac ruptured?
   b. Do you feel the urge to push?
   c. Are you having any vaginal discharge?
   d. How long were you in labor with the last child?

_____ **130.** After assessing the mother, you and your partner determine that she will most likely not deliver imminently, so you elect to initiate transport to the hospital, which is 25 miles away. Positioning of the patient in the left lateral recumbent position is important because
a. she will be facing you instead of the ambulance wall.
b. most pregnant patients find this position to be most comfortable.
c. it will relieve pressure off of the aorta, which could lower her cardiac output.
d. it will relieve pressure off of the inferior vena cava and maintain cardiac output.

_____ **131.** What other actions should you take during transport of this patient to the hospital?
a. Apply 100% supplemental oxygen.
b. Initiate two large-bore IVs.
c. Perform an internal vaginal examination.
d. Elevate the mother's lower extremities.

_____ **132.** With an estimated time of arrival (ETA) to the hospital of approximately 15 minutes, the mother tells you that she feels a great deal of pressure at the perineum. You visualize the area and see the top of the baby's head crowning from the vaginal opening. Would should you do FIRST?
a. Set up the OB kit for an imminent delivery.
b. Ensure that the mother is in the delivery position.
c. Time the interval and duration of her contractions.
d. Tell your partner to stop the ambulance immediately.

_____ **133.** A 16-year-old boy has a severe headache and vomiting that has progressively worsened over the past 36 hours. Which of the following questions would be MOST important to ask him?
a. Do you have a history of hypertension?
b. Have you experienced a recent head injury?
c. Do you have any abdominal pain or diarrhea?
d. Is there a history of meningitis in your family?

_____ **134.** Which of the following age groups BEST defines a toddler?
a. 6 to 12 months
b. 1 to 3 years
c. 3 to 5 years
d. 5 to 6 years

_____ **135.** Which of the following signs would you be MOST likely to see in a 2-month-old infant with a fever?
a. Shivering
b. Bradypnea
c. Tachycardia
d. Skin mottling

_____ **136.** When assessing the pupils of a patient who sustained a head injury, you note that they are bilaterally dilated and nonreactive. What does this MOST likely indicate?
a. Increased intracranial pressure
b. Pressure on the oculomotor nerve
c. Damage to the hypothalamus
d. A normal condition for the patient

_____ **137.** After performing your initial assessment and management of an unconscious nontrauma patient, your next MOST appropriate step should be to
  a. initiate rapid transport.
  b. obtain a SAMPLE history.
  c. perform a rapid assessment.
  d. perform a detailed physical examination.

_____ **138.** What is the major physiologic difference between cyanide and carbon monoxide?
  a. Cyanide attaches to the hemoglobin molecule.
  b. Cyanide destroys the cells of the immune system.
  c. Carbon monoxide destroys the red blood cells.
  d. Carbon monoxide binds with the hemoglobin molecule.

_____ **139.** A 6-year-old boy was struck by a car while riding his bicycle. He has a blood pressure of 60 systolic, a weak pulse rate of 150 beats/min, and respirations of 30 breaths/min. When providing fluid replacement, how much volume should you administer per bolus?
  a. 200 mL
  b. 400 mL
  c. 500 mL
  d. 650 mL

_____ **140.** What portion of the brain regulates a person's level of consciousness?
  a. Cerebrum
  b. Cerebellum
  c. Medulla oblongata
  d. Reticular activating system

_____ **141.** When assessing a 20-year-old woman with bilateral lower abdominal quadrant pain, which of the following findings is MOST suggestive of an ectopic pregnancy?
  a. Light vaginal discharge
  b. Missed menstrual period
  c. Denial of contraception use
  d. Tachycardia and hypotension

_____ **142.** A 45-year-old man sustained an isolated stab wound to the upper left thigh during a bar fight. As you approach him, he is conscious and screaming in pain. You can see bright red blood spurting from the wound. What should you do FIRST?
  a. Secure a patent airway.
  b. Administer 100% oxygen.
  c. Control the bleeding immediately.
  d. Manually control the cervical spine.

_____ **143.** Which of the following signs/symptoms would you be LEAST likely to find in a 19-year-old woman with cystitis?
  a. Polyuria
  b. Dysuria
  c. Urinary urgency
  d. Dysmenorrhea

_____**144.** The baroreceptors in the aorta and carotid arteries are extremely sensitive to
   a. increases in arterial carbon dioxide.
   b. changes in arterial perfusion pressure.
   c. changes in the rate and strength of the heart.
   d. fluctuations in the level of arterial oxygen.

_____**145.** A 30-year-old unrestrained woman struck the steering wheel after being involved in a deceleration accident while traveling approximately 40 miles per hour. She reports pain to the midsternal area, which is point tender to palpation. She has a blood pressure of 100/60 mm Hg, an irregular pulse rate of 118 beats/min, and slightly shallow respirations of 26 breaths/min. The remainder of your assessment is unremarkable. On the basis of this information, you should suspect
   a. a flail chest.
   b. pericardial tamponade.
   c. myocardial contusion.
   d. esophageal injury.

_____**146.** When a patient is in a state of shock (hypoperfusion), the sympathetic nervous system, through the release of catecholamines, is going to attempt to compensate to protect which of the following structures?
   a. Brain
   b. Heart
   c. Liver
   d. Kidneys

_____**147.** During your initial assessment of a trauma patient, you note tachycardia, diaphoresis, and restlessness. Assuming that hypovolemia is present, which of the following initial management techniques would MOST effectively reduce the negative effects of internal blood loss?
   a. Administer 100% oxygen.
   b. Elevate the lower extremities.
   c. Initiate an IV of normal saline solution.
   d. Apply and inflate the PASG.

_____**148.** Which of the following BEST describes a critical incident defusing?
   a. A formal process that involves all personnel involved
   b. A formal process that is held no longer than 12 hours after the incident
   c. An informal process that is held within 24 hours of the incident
   d. An informal process that is held within 2 to 4 hours following the incident

_____**149.** What is the MOST appropriate dose of diphenhydramine for a patient who is experiencing a severe allergic reaction?
   a. 0.3 to 0.5 mg IM
   b. 0.3 to 0.5 mg SC
   c. 25 to 50 mg IV
   d. 25 to 50 mg IM

_____**150.** The ratio of red blood cells to plasma is referred to as
   a. the hematocrit.
   b. carboxyhemoglobin.
   c. a complete blood count.
   d. partial thromboplastin time.

_____**151.** Findings of increased parasympathetic tone, bradycardia, the shunting of blood, and hypotension MOST accurately describe:
   a. Cushing's reflex.
   b. diving reflex.
   c. Beck's reflex.
   d. Cullen's sign.

_____**152.** Who has the ultimate medical authority at the scene of a mass-casualty incident?
   a. Fire chief
   b. Lead paramedic
   c. Medical director
   d. Incident commander

_____**153.** A conscious but confused patient has left-sided hemiparesis, facial droop, dysarthria, and a dilated, nonreactive right pupil. What is the most likely diagnosis?
   a. Right-sided hemorrhagic stroke
   b. Right-sided ischemic stroke
   c. Left-sided ischemic stroke
   d. Left-sided hemorrhagic stroke

_____**154.** In addition to viral and bacterial infectious processes, which of the following could also cause fever in a child?
   a. Inflammation
   b. Acute asthma
   c. Stress or anxiety
   d. Ingestion of diazepam

_____**155.** Which of the following injuries would MOST likely result from a motorcycle striking a fixed object?
   a. Chest and abdominal trauma
   b. Tibia, fibula, and pelvic fractures
   c. Femur fractures and head injury
   d. Thoracic spine and femur fractures

_____**156.** A 4-year-old boy has a high fever and deep, rapid respirations. The child's mother states that she thinks her child got into the medicine cabinet. Which of the following medications has the child MOST likely ingested?
   a. Acetaminophen
   b. Aspirin
   c. Codeine
   d. Ibuprofen

_____ **157.** Which of the following organs would produce the MOST rapid blood loss following penetrating trauma to the abdomen?
a. Liver
b. Spleen
c. Kidney
d. Pancreas

_____ **158.** A 34-year-old man calls EMS because of a possible allergic reaction following a bee sting. On your arrival, the patient is semiconscious with stridorous respirations, a generalized rash, and swelling to the face and neck. He has a blood pressure of 70 by palpation, a thready pulse rate of 140 beats/min, and labored respirations of 36 breaths/min. Which of the following treatments is MOST appropriate for this patient?
a. Ventilation with a BVM device and 0.3 to 0.5 mg of epinephrine 1:10,000 SC
b. Endotracheal intubation and 0.3 to 0.5 mg of epinephrine 1:10,000 IV
c. Needle cricothyrotomy and 0.3 to 0.5 mg of epinephrine 1:1,000 SC
d. Blind nasal intubation and 3 to 5 mg of epinephrine 1:10,000 IV

_____ **159.** All of the following conditions would likely result in a jaundiced appearance of the skin EXCEPT
a. inflammation of the liver.
b. an overdose of acetaminophen.
c. chronic renal insufficiency.
d. subacute bacterial meningitis.

_____ **160.** Which of the following situations BEST describes a mass-casualty incident?
a. When at least half of the patients are obviously dead
b. When there are two critical patients and one ambulance
c. When there are three stable patients and two ambulances
d. When there are at least 10 patients and half of them are critical

_____ **161.** The normal partial pressure of oxygen in arterial blood should be
a. 35 to 45 mm Hg.
b. 60 to 80 mm Hg.
c. 80 to 100 mm Hg.
d. 100 to 120 mm Hg.

_____ **162.** Following delivery of an infant, you suction, warm, and position the newborn. The infant's pulse rate is 90 beats/min, so you initiate positive pressure ventilations. After approximately 30 seconds of assisted ventilations, the pulse rate remains at 90 beats/min. Which of the following actions would be MOST appropriate for you to take next?
a. Suction the newborn's mouth and nose again if needed.
b. Administer 0.1 mg/kg of naloxone via the umbilical vein.
c. Administer 0.5 to 1 mg/kg of 25% dextrose via the umbilical vein.
d. Perform endotracheal intubation and begin chest compressions.

_____ **163.** What type of trauma is associated with the highest morbidity and mortality rate in infants and children?
   a. Chest
   b. Head
   c. Abdominal
   d. Cervical spine

_____ **164.** Which of the following injuries would MOST likely result in obstructive shock?
   a. Pelvic fracture
   b. Crushed trachea
   c. Simple pneumothorax
   d. Pericardial tamponade

_____ **165.** When arterial oxygen levels in the body are low, chemoreceptors in the brain send messages to the diaphragm and intercostal muscles via the
   a. phrenic nerve.
   b. vagus nerve.
   c. brainstem.
   d. medulla.

_____ **166.** A 2-year-old child has received partial-thickness burns to the entire face and head as well as both anterior legs from a suspected case of abuse. What percentage of the total body surface area does this represent?
   a. 23%
   b. 25%
   c. 32%
   d. 37%

_____ **167.** During a cardiac arrest involving a 5-year-old child, you administer epinephrine via the endotracheal tube. Which of the following represents the MOST appropriate dose when given by this route?
   a. 0.1 mg/kg of a 1:10,000 solution
   b. 0.1 mL/kg of a 1:1,000 solution
   c. 0.1 mL/kg of a 1:10,000 solution
   d. 0.01 mg/kg of a 1:1,000 solution

_____ **168.** When administering crystalloid solutions to a patient in severe hypovolemic shock, it is important for you to remember that
   a. you must give 1 mL for every 3 mL of estimated blood loss.
   b. you should limit the total volume of crystalloid in the field to 5 L.
   c. crystalloids do not increase the blood's oxygen-carrying capacity.
   d. crystalloids contain proteins and stay in the vascular space longer.

_____ **169.** Which of the following statements regarding the critical incident stress debriefing (CISD) process is FALSE?
   a. It should occur as soon as possible after the incident has occurred.
   b. Only the people directly involved in the incident are in attendance.
   c. The session discusses enhancing your skills for future incidents.
   d. Counselors who provide coping techniques are critical to the process.

_____ **170.** Which of the following BEST describes the process of gas exchange in the lungs?
  a. The transfer of carbon dioxide from the alveoli into the bloodstream is facilitated by a process called diffusion.
  b. The gases exchanged in the lungs always move from an area of greater concentration to an area of lesser concentration.
  c. Blood that returns to the lungs from the right side of the heart has a slightly lower level of carbon dioxide than oxygen.
  d. The partial pressure of oxygen in the alveoli is typically between 40 and 50 torr at the end of a maximal inhalation.

_____ **171.** When placing a cardiac monitor on a 6-month-old infant who is in profound respiratory distress with lethargy and an oxygen saturation of 82%, you would MOST likely see which of the following cardiac rhythms?
  a. Tachycardia with aberrant complexes
  b. Bradycardia with or without heart block
  c. An accelerated idioventricular rhythm
  d. AV dissociation and tachycardia

_____ **172.** Which of the following patients would be the BEST candidate for reperfusion therapy with a fibrinolytic agent?
  a. A 59-year-old woman with a sudden, severe headache, projectile vomiting, and a blood pressure of 180/110 mm Hg
  b. A 64-year-old man with dysarthria, left-sided facial droop, and left-sided hemiplegia for the past hour
  c. A 70-year-old man who takes warfarin and has had confusion and unilateral hemiparesis for the past 2 hours
  d. An 80-year-old woman who underwent recent hip surgery and who has had confusion and aphasia for the past 2 hours

_____ **173.** Tidal volume is BEST defined as the
  a. volume of air moved in and out of the lungs each minute.
  b. maximum volume of air that the lungs can accommodate.
  c. residual volume of air in the lungs at the end of exhalation.
  d. volume of air moved in and out of the lungs per breath.

_____ **174.** Which of the following medications is classified as a tricyclic anti-depressant?
  a. Fluoxetine hydrochloride
  b. Nortriptyline hydrochloride
  c. Buspirone hydrochloride
  d. Midazolam

_____ **175.** Which of the following is a CORRECT statement regarding the anger stage of the grieving process?
   a. The patient's anger is typically contained within, with little evidence of his or her feelings.
   b. Anger of the patient, when faced with a terminal illness, is not a typical stage of grieving.
   c. Displaced anger is not a personal attack on the individual to whom it is directed.
   d. The anger stage is typically the last emotional outlet that the patient experiences.

_____ **176.** Obsessive-compulsive disorder falls under which of the following psychiatric categories?
   a. Schizophrenia
   b. Functional social disorder
   c. Generalized anxiety disorder
   d. Posttraumatic stress disorder

_____ **177.** When forming the general impression of a medical patient, which of the following would MOST likely indicate an altered mental state?
   a. You are rudely told by the patient to leave.
   b. You note that the patient is quietly crying.
   c. The patient's speech pattern is altered.
   d. The patient maintains hypervigilance of your presence.

_____ **178.** During a mass-casualty incident, personnel gather at a central point and are sent by the incident commander to various areas of the scene. This central point is referred to as the
   a. staging area.
   b. triage sector.
   c. command post.
   d. transport sector.

—————— **Questions 179 and 180 pertain to the same patient.**——————

_____ **179.** On entering the residence of an elderly man, he is sitting on the couch with his eyes closed. His respirations appear to be deep and rapid. What should you do FIRST?
   a. Take spinal precautions.
   b. Assess his mental status.
   c. Perform a jaw-thrust maneuver.
   d. Immediately move him to the floor.

_____ **180.** In the absence of bystanders or family members, which of the following would be MOST reliable in establishing this particular patient's medical history?
   a. Look in the patient's wallet.
   b. Call the patient's neighbor.
   c. Perform a detailed physical examination.
   d. Check inside the refrigerator.

Table 2-1

Practice Final Examination Blueprint

Subtest and # of Items	Questions in Subtest	Minimum Suggested Correct	
Airway and Breathing (30)	1–3, 18, 26, 27, 29, 30, 45, 52, 65–68, 71, 91, 99, 101–103, 108, 111, 116, 120, 123, 127, 161, 165, 170, 173	21	
Cardiology (35)	5, 9, 13, 20, 21, 24, 31–33, 46–50, 78, 79, 82–84, 88–90, 92–98, 100, 109, 110, 112–114	23	
Trauma (31)	6–8, 10, 11, 25, 35, 36, 54, 55, 72, 73, 77, 80, 81, 104, 105, 107, 117, 122, 136, 142, 144–147, 150, 155, 157, 164, 168	22	
Medical (29)	4, 16, 17, 34, 42, 43, 59, 60, 69, 70, 86, 118, 119,126, 133, 137, 138, 140, 149, 151, 153, 158, 159,172, 174, 176, 177, 179, 180	21	
Obstetrics and Pediatrics (28)	14, 15, 19, 37–39, 44, 51, 85, 87, 115, 128–132, 134, 135, 139, 141, 143, 154, 156, 162, 163, 166, 167, 171	20	
Operations (27)	12, 22, 23, 28, 40, 41, 53, 56–58, 61–64, 74–76,106, 121, 124, 125, 148, 152, 160, 169, 175, 178	19	
180 ITEMS		**126**	

The Paramedic Practical Examination

The practical examination is no doubt stressful for the candidate. This is usually because they do not know what to expect. To alleviate some of the stress and anxiety associated with the practical examination; this section will provide you with information on the twelve skills that comprise the National EMT-Paramedic practical examination.

In addition to providing you with the performance checklists, key information pertinent to each skill, helpful tips and hints, commonly made errors and how to best avoid them, and sample scenarios will be provided. The skills that comprise the National EMT-Paramedic practical examination are as follows:

1. Trauma Patient Assessment/Management

2. Adult Ventilatory Management
   • Endotracheal Intubation and,
   • Dual Lumen Airway Device (either the Combitube® or the PtL®)

3. Cardiac Management Skills
   • Dynamic Cardiology
   • Static Cardiology

4. Oral Station
   • Station A
   • Station B

5. IV and Medication Skills
- Intravenous Therapy
- Intravenous Bolus Medications

6. Pediatric Skills
- Pediatric (<2 years of age) Ventilatory Management
- Pediatric Intraosseous Infusion

7. Random Basic Skills (one of the following at random)
- Spinal Immobilization (seated patient)
- Spinal Immobilization (supine patient)
- Bleeding Control/Shock Management

Notice: The National Registry of EMT's has granted the author the right to reproduce the skill performance checklists contained within this manual, in whole or in part. The National Registry of EMT's is not responsible for the enhancements made to the skill checklists in this publication, nor do they endorse such enhancements.

Skill Station Examiners

The skill station examiners have been chosen based upon their expertise in the skill in which they will be evaluating. They will serve as objective recorders of your actions and will provide you with all information necessary to perform the skill. Keep in mind that some skill examiners document more than others. The amount of documentation does not indicate your level of performance in the skill station. Remain focused on what you are doing, not what the examiner is writing or not writing. On completion of a skill, the examiner is not allowed to give you feedback or in any way indicate your degree of performance. The skill examiner is unaware of the minimum point values that must be met for each skill. This further ensures their maximum objectivity in recording your performance.

The Performance Checklists

The performance checklists for each of the paramedic skills represent a logical fashion in which to perform the skill. Many candidates focus on literally memorizing the sequence of the skill performance checklist instead of concentrating on and understanding the events that must occur within that sequence.

When preparing for the practical examination, it is clearly smart to be thoroughly familiar with the performance checklist however; a healthy understanding of the concept and objectives of the skill is far more vital. Just because you miss a few steps in a particular skill does not equate to automatic failure. The reason why candidates do not successfully complete a skill is because they perform actions or fail to perform actions that would result in harm to the patient or themselves. These actions or inactions are what comprise the established critical criteria for each skill.

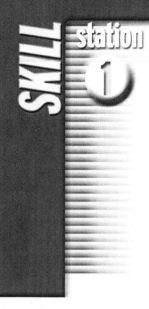
Trauma Patient Assessment/Management

Station Time Limit: 10 minutes.

Skill Station Objective: You will be required to perform an assessment on a live moulaged trauma patient and verbalize the management for all conditions and injuries that you discover. You must conduct the assessment just as you would in a real-life field situation, to include communicating with your patient. As you progress through the skill, you must state everything that you are assessing.

Your Partner(s): You will have two "phantom" partners working with you that are trained to your level of care. Your partners will correctly perform the verbal treatments that you request.

Skill Examiner Function(s): The skill station examiner will provide specific clinical information not obtainable by visual or physical assessment. An example would be providing you with the patient's vital signs but only if you ask for them. The examiner will not provide you with information not contained in the scenario unless you ask for it. At times, the examiner may ask you for additional information if clarification is needed. For example, if you state that you are placing the patient on "high-flow oxygen," the examiner would ask you how you would accomplish that.

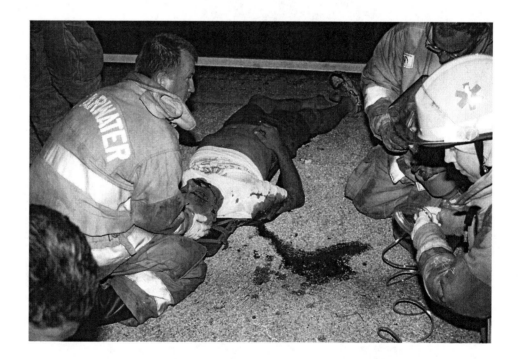

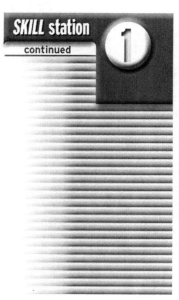

SKILL station
continued
1

Table 3-1

Trauma Patient Assessment Performance Checklist

Trauma Patient Assessment			
Takes or verbalizes body substance isolation precautions	1		
SCENE SIZE-UP			
Determines the scene/situation is safe	1		
Determines the mechanism of injury/nature of illness	1		
Determines the number of patients	1		
Requests additional help if necessary	1		
Considers stabilization of the spine	1		
INITIAL ASSESSMENT/RESUSCITATION			
Verbalizes general impression of the patient	1		
Determines responsiveness/level of consciousness	1		
Determines chief complaint/apparent life threats	1		
Airway Opens and assesses airway (1 point)—Inserts adjunct as indicated (1 point)	2		
Breathing -Assesses breathing (1 point) -Ensures adequate ventilation (1 point) -Initiates appropriate oxygen therapy (1 point) -Manages any injury which may compromise breathing/ventilation (1 point)	4		
Circulation -Checks pulse (1 point) -Assess skin [either skin color, temperature, or condition] (1 point) -Assesses for and controls major bleeding if present (1 point) -Initiates shock management (1 point)	4		
Identifies priority patients/makes transport decision	1		
FOCUSED HISTORY AND PHYSICAL EXAMINATION/RAPID TRAUMA ASSESSMENT			
Selects appropriate assessment	1		
Obtains or directs assistant to obtain baseline vital signs	1		
Obtains SAMPLE history	1		
DETAILED PHYSICAL EXAMINATION			
Head -Inspects mouth, nose, and assesses facial area (1 point) -Inspects and palpates scalp and ears (1 point) -Assesses eyes for PEARRL (1 point)	3		
Neck -Checks position of trachea (1 point) -Checks jugular veins (1 point) -Palpates cervical spine (1 point)	3		
Chest -Inspects chest (1 point) -Palpates chest (1 point) -Auscultates chest (1 point)	3		
Abdomen/pelvis -Inspects and palpates abdomen (1 point) -Assesses pelvis (1 point) -Verbalizes assessment of genitalia/perineum as needed (1 point)	3		

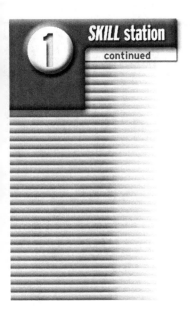

Trauma Patient Assessment (continued)

Lower extremities -Inspects, palpates, and assesses motor, sensory, and distal circulation functions (1 point/leg)	2	
Upper extremities -Inspects, palpates, and assesses motor, sensory, and distal circulation functions (1 point/arm)	2	
Posterior thorax, lumbar, and buttocks -Inspects and palpates posterior thorax (1 point) -Inspects and palpates lumbar and buttocks area (1 point)	2	
Manages secondary injuries and wounds appropriately	1	
Performs ongoing assessment	1	
Modeled from the NREMT Performance Skill Sheet	43	

To best prepare for this skill station, you should review the patient assessment and trauma sections of your paramedic textbook and practice frequently while following the steps of the performance checklist (Table 3-1). If you have recently taken courses such as Basic Trauma Life Support (BTLS) or Prehospital Trauma Life Support (PHTLS), you should be well prepared for this station.

Remember that this is not an evaluation exclusive of your ability to assess a trauma patient. You must integrate the appropriate management within your assessment as well.

The vast majority of errors made during this station center around the candidate focusing more on the assessment and less on providing the appropriate management at the appropriate time. Just as you would on a real call, you must provide immediate care for all life-threatening injuries as soon as you discover them (ie, inadequate breathing, altered mental status, severe bleeding, etc).

Critical Criteria: Trauma Patient Assessment/Management

1. **Failure to initiate or call for transport of the patient within a 10-minute time limit.**
   - Remember that this station, with the exception of the actual "hands-on assess-ment," is completely verbalized. If you do not verbally inform the examiner that you are physically in the back of the ambulance and en route to the hospital, he/she will not record you as such.
   - Transport should occur as soon as you have completed the rapid trauma assess-ment, managed all immediate life threats, and verbalized full spinal precautions.

2. **Failure to take or verbalize body substance isolation precautions.**
   - This is such an easy task, yet it is frequently forgotten. To avoid falling into that trap, physically place gloves on your hands prior to entering the station.

3. **Failure to determine scene safety.**
   - There is no trick or tip to prompt you to remember this critical step. Just keep one thought in mind; the life you save may take your own! Treat this skill station with the same respect for safety that you would in a real life situation.

4. **Failure to assess for and provide spinal protection when indicated.**
   - Do not focus on the "when indicated" part of this critical criteria. It is indicated because you are dealing with a critical trauma patient; therefore, spinal injury is assumed.
   - Do not speak to the patient until you have directed your partner to manually stabilize the patient's head.

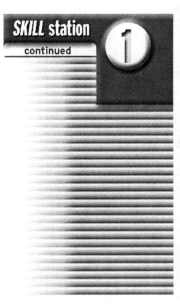

5. Failure to voice and ultimately provide a high concentration of oxygen.
- Remember, trauma patients receive oxygen in one of two forms; either with a nonrebreathing mask at 15 L/min or attached to a BVM device when assisting ventilations.
- Do not forget to verbalize to the examiner that whichever method of oxygen delivery you use, 100% oxygen is attached.

6. Failure to assess/provide adequate ventilation.
- Remember that simple concept of ABC? Do not negate assessment of the patient's respirations based on the premise that he/she will need a nonrebreathing mask. A nonrebreathing mask on a patient with shallow respirations at a rate of 8 breaths/min is NOT appropriate airway management.
- If in doubt as to the adequacy of the patient's breathing, err on the side of providing ventilations. The worst thing that can happen is that the examiner states that the patient will not allow it.
- *At a minimum,* the patient must be on a nonrebreathing mask at 15 L/min.

7. Failure to find or appropriately manage problems associated with airway, breathing, hemorrhage, or shock [hypoperfusion].
- Remember the flow of this station: find it, fix it, and continue assessing.
- If you perform a systematic, methodical assessment, you will not leave anything out. You must find an injury in order to fix it.
- DO NOT focus strictly on assessing the patient. Manage all immediate life threats on discovery. These tasks can be delegated to your "phantom" partners.
- Do not forget to initiate basic shock management in the initial assessment, such as keeping the patient warm and elevating the lower extremities.
- Here are some examples of immediate life threats, where in the assessment you would be most likely to discover them, and how to appropriately manage them.
  - Initial Assessment Findings
    - *Secretions in the airway:* Immediate suction prior to providing the appropriate ventilatory support.
    - *Injuries that compromise the airway (ie, airway swelling, massive airway trauma, etc):* This situation may require immediate intubation.
    - *Apnea/Inadequate breathing:* Initiate positive pressure ventilations. Insert an oral or nasal airway if indicated. Otherwise, apply a nonrebreathing mask at 15 L/min. Consider intubation provided that it does not delay your assessment and transport.
    - *Major bleeding:* Delegate your partner to immediately control the bleeding.
    - *Signs of shock (ie, absent peripheral pulses, diaphoresis, rapid and shallow breathing, etc):* You must immediately initiate basic shock treatment as mentioned above.
  - Rapid Trauma Assessment Findings
    - *Recheck airway and breathing:* Manage any new problems that may have developed.
    - *Tension pneumothorax:* Immediate needle decompression in between the second and third intercostal space, mid-clavicular line.
    - *Flail chest:* Immediate hand stabilization, followed by stabilization with a bulky dressing (no sandbags).
    - *Sucking chest wound:* Immediately seal the wound with an occlusive dressing and continually monitor for a potentially developing tension pneumothorax.
    - *Abdominal evisceration:* Immediately cover with a moist, sterile dressing, covered with a dry, sterile dressing.
    - *Unstable pelvis:* Do not logroll the patient. Use a scoop and place the patient on the spineboard. Consider stabilizing with the PASG. Do not repalpate in the detailed physical examination.

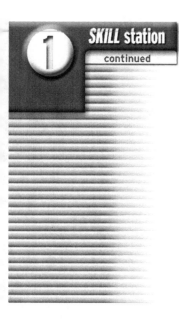

- *Bilateral femur fractures:* Do not logroll the patient. Use a scoop and place the patient on the spineboard. Consider stabilizing with the PASG. Do not repalpate in the detailed physical examination.

8. Failure to differentiate patient's need for immediate transportation versus continued assessment/treatment at the scene.

- ANY problems with airway, breathing, or circulation as well as signs and/or symptoms of shock will require immediate transport.
- This critical element is commonly checked because the candidate failed to verbally inform the examiner that they were en route to the hospital so when the detailed physical examination began, the examiner assumed that the candidate was still at the scene and not in the ambulance.

9. Performs other detailed/focused history or physical examination before assessing/treating threats to airway, breathing, and circulation.

- Remember, ALL patients must have an initial assessment first. Problems with the ABCs will kill a patient before anything else, no matter how obvious or grotesque.
- Candidates will frequently see obvious injuries and tend to focus on them first. Avoid tunnel vision on the obvious injuries for it is the obvious that is usually the least life threatening.

10. Orders a dangerous or inappropriate procedure.

- This is where your judgment is going to play a key role in your performance. If you are unsure of whether or not a particular procedure is required, it is best NOT to perform the procedure and continue to manage the overall situation (ie, shock, inadequate breathing, etc). Keep in mind this general information to avoid making a dangerous decision:
  - Trauma patients, unless in cardiac arrest, rarely require any form of medication therapy other than oxygen.
  - Never logroll a patient with an unstable pelvis. Use a scoop stretcher instead.
  - Remember that once you perform a procedure, you cannot take it back. Make 100% sure that it is indicated.
  - Use the PASG for pelvic fractures and bilateral femur fractures. Traction splints take too long to apply.
  - The vest-style device (ie, KED) is not appropriate for a critical trauma patient.
  - Prioritize your management based on *what is going to kill the patient first.*

Adult Ventilatory Management

During this station, you will be required to demonstrate the correct techniques for endotracheal intubation **and** one of the two dual lumen airway devices, either the Combitube, **or** the Pharyngeal Tracheal Lumen (PtL) airway devices.

Both of these airway skills are typically tested in the same station, by the same examiner. You will not be required to place the endotracheal (ET) tube and then place one of the two dual lumen devices around the ET tube. They are tested as two different procedures.

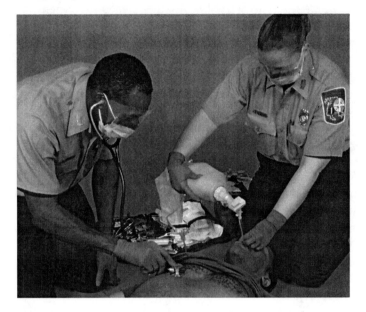

Skill 2A: Adult Endotracheal Intubation

Station Time Limit: There is no set time limit for this station.

Skill Station Objective: This skill is designed to evaluate your ability to provide immediate and aggressive ventilatory assistance to an apneic adult with a pulse who has no injuries. This is a nontrauma situation, so cervical precautions are not necessary. You are required to demonstrate sequentially all procedures you would perform, from simple maneuvers and adjuncts to endotracheal intubation. You will have three attempts to successfully intubate the manikin. You must actually ventilate the manikin for at least 30 seconds with each adjunct and procedure used.

Your Partner(s): The skill examiner will serve as your trained assistant and will be interacting with you throughout this skill. He/she will correctly carry out your orders on your direction.

Skill Examiner Function(s): In addition to recording your actions, the skill examiner will serve as your trained assistant. You will be provided 2 minutes to check your equipment and prepare whatever you feel is necessary.

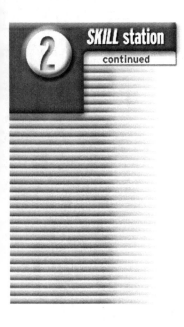

Table 3-2

Adult Endotracheal Intubation Performance Checklist

Adult Ventilatory Management: Endotracheal Intubation		
Takes or verbalizes body substance isolation precautions	1	
Opens the airway manually	1	
Elevates tongue, inserts simple adjunct [oropharyngeal or nasopharyngeal airway]	1	
Note: Examiner now informs candidate no gag reflex is present and patient accepts adjunct.		
Ventilates patient immediately with BVM device unattached to oxygen	1	
Ventilates patient with room air	1	
Note: Examiner now informs candidate that ventilation is being performed without difficulty and that pulse oximetry indicates the patient's blood oxygen saturation is 85%.		
Attaches oxygen reservoir to BVM device and connects to high-flow oxygen regulator [12 to 15 L/min]	1	
Ventilates patient at a rate of 10 to 12/min with appropriate volumes	1	
Note: After 30 seconds, examiner auscultates and reports breath sounds are present, equal bilaterally, and medical control has ordered intubation. The examiner must now take over ventilation.		
Directs assistant to pre-oxygenate patient	1	
Identifies/selects proper equipment for intubation	1	
Checks equipment for: -Cuff leaks (1 point) -Laryngoscope operational with bulb tight (1 point)	2	
Note: Examiner to remove OPA and move out of the way when candidate is prepared to intubate.		
Positions head properly	1	
Inserts blade while displacing tongue	1	
Elevates mandible with laryngoscope	1	
Introduces ET tube and advances to proper depth	1	
Inflates cuff to proper pressure and disconnects syringe	1	
Confirms proper placement by auscultation bilaterally over each lung and over epigastrium as the patient is being ventilated	1	
Note: Examiner to ask "If you had proper placement, what should you expect to hear?"		
Secures ET tube (may be verbalized)	1	
Note: Examiner now asks candidate, "Please demonstrate one additional method of verifying proper tube placement in this patient."		
Identifies/selects proper equipment	1	
Verbalizes findings and interpretations [compares indicator color to the colorimetric scale or EDD recoil and states findings]	1	
Note: Examiner now states, "You see secretions in the tube and hear gurgling sounds with the patient's exhalations."		
Identifies/selects a flexible suction catheter	1	
Pre-oxygenates patient	1	
Marks maximum insertion length with thumb and forefinger	1	
Inserts catheter into ET tube leaving catheter port open	1	
At proper insertion depth, covers catheter port and applies suction while withdrawing catheter	1	
Ventilates/directs ventilation of patient as catheter is flushed with sterile water	1	
Modeled from the NREMT Performance Skill Sheet	27	

This skill station generally is not too problematic for most candidates. Those who do not successfully complete on the first attempt usually did so because they took too long to intubate the manikin (greater than 30 seconds) or were not able to successfully intubate within three attempts. This was typically the result of their lack of familiarization with the particular manikin at the test site. If at all possible, practice on several different types of manikins as some are more difficult to intubate than others.

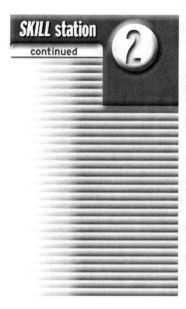

SKILL station
continued

Critical Criteria: Adult Endotracheal Intubation

1. Failure to initiate ventilations within 30 seconds after applying gloves or interrupts ventilations for greater than 30 seconds at any time.
   - Remember, you have 2 minutes to prepare whatever equipment you think is necessary. It would be wise to fully assemble the BVM device if it is not already assembled. Also, get your oral airways in place so that they are easily accessible when you begin.
   - Thirty seconds may seem like a long time, but it can fly by if you are not keeping track of your time. There is no shame in counting out loud; 1 1,000, 2 1,000, 3 1,000, etc.

2. Failure to take or verbalize body substance isolation precautions.
   - As with all skills, if you physically walk into the station with gloves on, you are covered. Even though critical criteria #1 states that you must begin ventilations within 30 seconds after applying gloves, you still have 2 minutes to set up your equipment.

3. Failure to voice and ultimately provide a high oxygen concentration [at least 85%].
   - Initially in the station, you can either ventilate the patient with room air or begin ventilations with the BVM device already connected to 100% oxygen and the reservoir attached. In your setup time, it is suggested that you fully assemble the BVM device and have it prepared to deliver 100% oxygen. Just remember to verbally inform the examiner that the BVM device is attached to supplemental oxygen with the flowmeter set at 15 L/min.

4. Failure to ventilate the patient at a rate of at least 10 to 12/min.
   - Ensure that no matter what, you ventilate at least once every 5 to 6 seconds, which will ensure at least 10 to 12 ventilations per minute. Again, there is no shame in counting out loud. It beats having to repeat the station. The examiner will be timing you.

5. Failure to provide adequate volumes per breath [maximum 2 errors/min are permissible].
   - Remember that the most difficult part of using a BVM device with one person is to maintain an effective seal, especially if you have small hands. Practice using the c-clamp method to ensure that effective volume is delivered per breath. As long as the chest is rising well, you are providing effective ventilation.
   - Inquire about taking a pocket mask into the station (must be cleared with the NREMT representative first). Recall from the performance checklist that the *initial* ventilations can be provided with room air. It is much easier to provide good tidal volume with a pocket mask. Once the patient is *successfully* intubated, you will have no trouble providing adequate volume.

6. Failure to pre-oxygenate the patient prior to intubating and suctioning.
   - After you have provided a period of ventilation with 100% oxygen, the examiner then assumes the role of your partner. Remember to verbally inform them to pre-oxygenate the patient as you are assembling your intubation equipment.
   - Make sure that you had preassembled the BVM device to include the attachment of a reservoir and supplemental oxygen at 15 L/min. The examiner will NOT remind you of this.

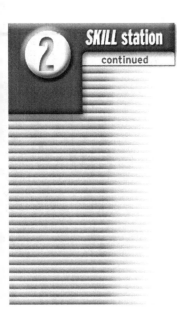

SKILL station
continued

7. Failure to successfully intubate within three attempts.

- As previously mentioned, most candidates have trouble intubating because they are not used to practicing with the type of manikin that may be used at the test site. Practice with several different types.
- NEVER advance the ET tube until you have visualized the vocal cords. The best initial indicator of successful tube placement is when you visualize the tube passing in between the cords. A "blind" intubation will undoubtedly end up in the hypopharyngeal space (the esophagus).
- Don't forget to keep track of your time during your intubation attempt(s). You cannot interrupt ventilations for greater than 30 seconds at any time.

8. Failure to disconnect syringe immediately after inflating the cuff of the ET tube.

- In your 2-minute setup time, preconnect the syringe to the ET tube. When you grab the tube to attempt intubation, hold the syringe (already attached to the pilot balloon of the tube) against the tube. After the tube is in place and you reach for the BVM device, the first thing you will see is the syringe dangling from the tube. This will serve as a good prompt to inflate the cuff with 5 to 10 mL of air and immediately remove the syringe.

9. Uses teeth as a fulcrum.

- Using the proper technique with the laryngoscope easily prevents this. NEVER pry with the handle. Lift with the long axis of the handle instead.
- A technique that you might try is to place your left forearm (remember, intubation is a left-handed technique) on the forehead of the manikin as your elbow rests on the table. This will greatly increase the amount of leverage that you have and minimize the risk of prying.

10. Failure to ensure proper tube placement by auscultating bilaterally and over the epigastrium.

- The new AHA verbiage is "5-point auscultation." Have the stethoscope hanging around your neck as you are progressing through this station. This is a good prompt to remember to auscultate.
- Remember, you must first inflate and immediately remove the syringe.

11. If used, stylet extends beyond the end of the ET tube.

- In your preparation time, make sure that the stylet is receded at least 2 cm from the distal end of the tube. The stylet should come to rest at the proximal portion of Murphy's eye (the hole in the distal side of the tube).
- After placing the stylet, bend the proximal end over the ET tube to prevent it from slipping.

12. Inserts any adjunct in a manner that is dangerous to the patient.

- Remember to correctly size the oral airway prior to placing it to ensure the most appropriate size. You must also demonstrate the correct placement procedure.
- Prelubricate both the ET tube and the mouth of the manikin to facilitate an easier intubation. You do not want to have to force the tube into place, which may give the examiner the impression that you are being too rough.
- When you suction, remember to suction on the way out.

13. Suctions the patient for more than 10 seconds.

- Play it safe, count out loud to yourself as you suction the patient and limit suction time to 10 seconds.

14. Does not suction the patient.

- When the examiner mentions the word "gurgling," think suction. You know as well as any body else that continuing to ventilate the patient with thick tracheal secretions will cause harm to the patient (increased hypoxia).

Skill 2B: Dual Lumen Airway Devices

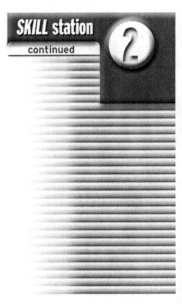

SKILL station
continued
2

Station Time Limit: There is no set time limit for this station.

Skill Station Objective: This skill is designed to evaluate your ability to provide immediate and aggressive ventilatory assistance to an apneic patient with a pulse who has no injuries. This is a nontrauma situation, so cervical precautions are not necessary. You are required to demonstrate sequentially all procedures you would perform, from simple maneuvers and adjuncts to placement of a dual lumen airway device of your choosing. You will have three attempts to successfully place the Combitube or PtL. You must actually ventilate the manikin for at least 30 seconds with each adjunct and procedure used.

Your Partner(s): The skill examiner will serve as your trained assistant and will be interacting with you throughout these skills. He/she will correctly carry out your orders on your direction.

Skill Examiner Function(s): In addition to recording your actions, the skill examiner will serve as your trained assistant. You will be provided 2 minutes to check your equipment and prepare whatever you feel is necessary.

Table 3-3

Dual Lumen Airway Device Performance Checklist

Adult Ventilatory Management: Dual Lumen Airway Device		
Takes or verbalizes body substance isolation precautions	1	
Opens the airway manually	1	
Elevates tongue, inserts simple adjunct [oropharyngeal or nasopharyngeal airway]	1	
Note: Examiner now informs candidate no gag reflex is present and patient accepts adjunct.		
Ventilates patient immediately with BVM device unattached to oxygen	1	
Ventilates patient with room air	1	
Note: Examiner now informs candidate that ventilation is being performed without difficulty.		
Attaches oxygen reservoir to BVM device and connects to high-flow oxygen regulator [12 to 15 L/min]	1	
Ventilates patient at a rate of 10 to 12/min with appropriate volumes	1	
Note: After 30 seconds, examiner auscultates and reports breath sounds are present, equal bilaterally, and medical control has ordered insertion of a dual lumen airway. The examiner must now take over ventilation.		
Directs assistant to pre-oxygenate patient	1	
Checks/prepares airway device	1	
Lubricates distal tip of the device [may be verbalized]	1	
Note: Examiner to remove OPA and move out of the way when candidate is prepared to insert device.		
Positions head properly	1	
Performs a tongue-jaw lift	1	

SKILL station
continued

Adult Ventilatory Management: Dual Lumen Airway Device (continued)			
Uses Combitube	Uses PtL		
Inserts device in midline and to depth so printed ring is at level of teeth	Inserts device in midline until bite block flange is at level of teeth	1	
Inflates pharyngeal cuff with proper volume and removes syringe	Secures strap	1	
Inflates distal cuff with proper volume and removes syringe	Blows into tube #1 to adequately inflate both cuffs	1	
Attaches/directs attachment of BVM device to the first [esophageal placement] lumen and ventilates		1	
Confirms placement and ventilation through correct lumen by observing chest rise, auscultation over the epigastrium, and bilaterally over each lung		1	
Note: The examiner states, "You do not see rise and fall of the chest and you only hear sounds over the epigastrium."			
Attaches/directs attachment of BVM device to the second [endotracheal placement] lumen and ventilates		1	
Confirms placement and ventilation through correct lumen by observing chest rise, auscultation over the epigastrium, and bilaterally over each lung		1	
Note: The examiner confirms adequate chest rise, absent sounds over the epigastrium, and equal bilateral breath sounds.			
Secures device or confirms that the device remains properly secured		1	
Modeled from the NREMT Performance Skill Sheet		20	

The vast majority of candidates that do not successfully complete this phase of the ventilatory management station were simply not familiar with the devices. In preparation for this skill, it would clearly behoove the candidate to obtain both of the dual lumen airway devices and practice with them until they feel comfortable with both.

The site coordinator must have both devices present. This will allow you to choose the device that you are most comfortable with and elect to use that one for testing.

Critical Criteria: Dual Lumen Airway Device

1. **Failure to initiate ventilations within 30 seconds after applying gloves or interrupts ventilations for greater than 30 seconds at any time.**
   - Remember, you have 2 minutes to prepare whatever equipment you think is necessary. It would be wise to fully assemble the BVM device if it is not already assembled. Also, get your oral airways in place so that they are easily accessible when you begin.
   - Thirty seconds may seem like a long time, but it can fly by if you are not keeping track of your time. There is no shame in counting out loud; 1 1,000, 2 1,000, 3 1,000, etc.
2. **Failure to take or verbalize body substance isolation precautions.**
   - As with all skills, if you walk into the station with gloves on, you are covered. Even though critical criteria #1 states that you must begin ventilations within 30 seconds after applying gloves, you still have 2 minutes to set up your equipment.

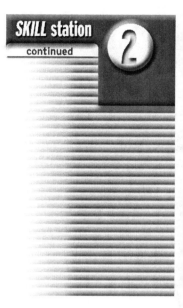

3. **Failure to voice and ultimately provide a high oxygen concentration [at least 85%].**
    - Initially in the station, you can either ventilate the patient with room air or begin ventilations with the BVM device already connected to 100% oxygen and the reservoir attached. In your setup time, it is suggested that you fully assemble the BVM device and have it prepared to deliver 100% oxygen. Just remember to verbally inform the examiner that the BVM device is attached to supplemental oxygen with the flowmeter set at 15 L/min.

4. **Failure to ventilate the patient at a rate of at least 10 to 12/min.**
    - Ensure that no matter what, you ventilate at least once every 5 to 6 seconds, which will ensure at least 10 to 12 ventilations per minute. Again, there is no shame in counting out loud. It beats having to repeat the station. The examiner will be timing you.

5. **Failure to provide adequate volumes per breath [maximum 2 errors/min are permissible].**
    - Remember that the most difficult part of using a BVM device with one person is to maintain an effective seal, especially if you have small hands. Practice using the c-clamp method to ensure that effective volume is delivered per breath. As long as the chest is rising well, you are providing effective ventilation.
    - Inquire about taking a pocket mask into the station. Recall from the performance checklist that the *initial* ventilations can be provided with room air. It is much easier to provide good tidal volume with a pocket mask. Once the patient is *successfully* intubated, you will have no trouble providing adequate volume.

6. **Failure to pre-oxygenate prior to insertion of the dual lumen airway device.**
    - After you have provided a period of ventilation with 100% oxygen, the examiner then assumes the role of your partner. Remember to verbally inform them to pre-oxygenate the patient as you are assembling your intubation equipment.
    - Make sure that you had pre-assembled the BVM device to include the attachment of a reservoir and supplemental oxygen at 15 L/min. The examiner will NOT remind you of this.

7. **Failure to insert dual lumen airway device at a proper depth or proper place within three attempts.**
    - With the Combitube, the depth markings (black rings on the tube) should be between the patient's teeth.
    - With the PtL, the bite block flange must be at the level of the teeth.
    - Use the tongue-jaw lift when inserting both devices. The correct head position for both the Combitube and the PtL should be in the neutral position.

8. **Failure to inflate both cuffs properly.**
    - The pharyngeal cuff (large proximal cuff) of the Combitube must be inflated with 100 mL of air and the distal cuff inflated with 5 to 10 mL.
    - Do not forget to disconnect the syringe from the cuff inflation valve when using the Combitube.
    - With the PtL, blow into the inflation valve (the larger of the two) with a sustained breath until you meet resistance against your breath. This is a one-way valve that does not require a syringe.

9. **Combitube—Failure to remove the syringe immediately after inflation of each cuff.**
    - In your 2-minute setup time, preconnect the syringe to the Combitube. When you grab the tube to attempt intubation, hold the syringe (already attached to the pilot balloon of the tube) against the tube. After the tube is in place and you reach for the BVM device, the first thing you will see is the syringe dangling from the tube. This will serve as a good prompt to inflate both cuffs and immediately remove the syringe.

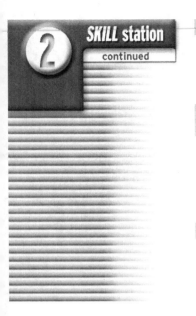

10. **PtL—Failure to secure the strap prior to cuff inflation.**
- Unlike the Combitube, whose large pharyngeal cuff secures the tube in place when inflated, the pharyngeal cuff on the PtL is inflated with much less air and will not serve to adequately secure the device; therefore, the strap must be secured prior to inflation of *both* cuffs.

11. **Failure to confirm that the proper lumen of the device is being ventilated by observing chest rise, auscultation over the epigastrium, and bilaterally over each lung.**
- Remember, you will ventilate through the lumen that produces chest rise and audible breath sounds. Since this is a blind technique, the tube will come to rest in the esophagus the majority of the time.
- Have the stethoscope hanging around your neck as you are progressing through this station. This is a good prompt to remember to auscultate.

12. **Inserts any adjunct in a manner that is dangerous to the patient.**
- Remember to correctly size the oral airway prior to placing it to ensure the most appropriate size. You must also demonstrate the correct placement procedure.
- Prelubricate whichever dual lumen device you will be using and the mouth of the manikin to facilitate an easier intubation. You do not want to have to force the device into place, which may give the examiner the impression that you are being too rough.

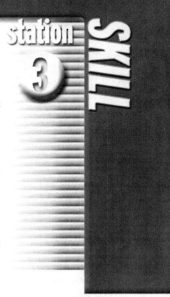

Skill Station 3: Cardiac Management Skills

The cardiac management station is comprised of two skills, dynamic and static cardiology, which is typically tested within the same station by the same examiner. We will look at the dynamic cardiology station first, which is identical to the "Megacode" that you either practiced in class or have encountered in an ACLS course. The static cardiology station is likened to the "Therapeutic Modalities" station of an ACLS course. All management performed within this station **must** adhere to the 2005 American Heart Association Guidelines and Algorithms.

Note: Just as it sometimes occurs in the field, some patients do not respond favorably despite appropriate management. The patient's response in the prepared scenarios presented to you is not meant to give any indication whatsoever as to your performance in this skill.

Skill 3A: Dynamic Cardiology

Station Time Limit: 8 minutes.

Skill Station Objective: This skill is designed to evaluate your ability to recognize and treat cardiac arrhythmias in accordance with current American Heart Association guidelines and algorithms. In the dynamic cardiology station, you will be evaluated using the defibrillation manikin and ECG monitor/defibrillator. Four separate arrhythmias will be presented in which you must act as the team leader and voice your interpretation of each arrhythmia as well as all basic and advanced life support and pharmacological interventions necessary throughout this skill. Please leave the defibrillator turned down to its lowest energy setting and verbally state the actual energy level that you would be delivering to the patient if this were an actual event. You must physically demonstrate the correct use of the defibrillator, including switching leads and performing actual defibrillation using correct paddle placement.

Your Partner(s): You will have "phantom" partners who will correctly provide the appropriate management that you direct them to.

Skill Examiner Function(s): The skills examiner will record your actions, monitor your time limit, and provide you with the arrhythmias, using a rhythm generator, that you will be expected to manage. Additionally, the examiner will give you a few moments to familiarize yourself with the equipment and will explain any of the specific operational features of the monitor/defibrillator.

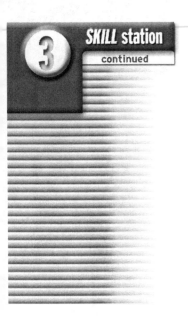

Table 3-4

Dynamic Cardiology Performance Checklist

Dynamic Cardiology		
Takes or verbalizes infection control precautions	1	
Checks level of responsiveness	1	
Checks ABCs	1	
Initiates CPR when appropriate [verbally]	1	
Attaches ECG monitor in a timely fashion [pads or paddles]	1	
Correctly interprets initial rhythm	1	
Appropriately manages initial rhythm	2	
Notes change in rhythm	1	
Checks patient condition to include pulse and, if appropriate, BP	1	
Correctly interprets second rhythm	1	
Appropriately manages second rhythm	2	
Notes change in rhythm	1	
Checks patient condition to include pulse and, if appropriate, BP	1	
Correctly interprets third rhythm	1	
Appropriately manages third rhythm	2	
Notes change in rhythm	1	
Checks patient condition to include pulse and, if appropriate, BP	1	
Correctly interprets fourth rhythm	1	
Appropriately manages fourth rhythm	2	
Orders high percentage of supplemental oxygen at proper times	1	
Modeled from the NREMT Performance Skill Sheet	**24**	

If you have recently taken an ACLS course and successfully completed the Megacode, you should not have a problem with the dynamic cardiology station. With the exception of physically demonstrating the correct use of the defibrillator paddles, this station is completely verbalized. You will be presented with an initial scenario and will then be expected to provide the most appropriate patient management.

Note that the scenario in which you will be presented may or may not begin with a patient in cardiac arrest. The patient may be conscious and have severe chest pain. The flow of the scenario is preset and should not be construed as an indicator of your performance.

There are a variety of scenarios that you might be presented with. If you follow the current ACLS guidelines and use a systematic and methodical approach, just like you did in the patient assessment station, you should not have any problems with this station. Just remember that this is a dynamic station that will require you to "adjust fire" and change algorithms midstream.

Critical Criteria: Dynamic Cardiology

1. Failure to deliver any shock in a timely manner.

- The best way to avoid this mistake is by using the quick-look feature on the monitor/defibrillator. Attaching the leads takes too much time and will result in an unnecessary delay in defibrillation.
- Remember that if the patient presents in either ventricular fibrillation or pulseless ventricular tachycardia, *defibrillation takes priority over all else.*

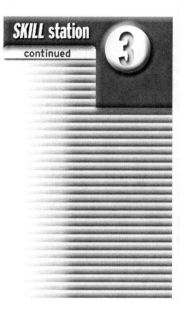

SKILL station
continued
3

2. **Failure to verify rhythm before delivering each shock.**
   - When you look at the monitor to assess the rhythm, be sure that you verbalize your interpretation to the examiner.
   - The examiner will not assume that you know that the rhythm is ventricular fibrillation simply because you defibrillate.

3. **Failure to ensure the safety of self and others [verbalizes "All Clear" and observes].**
   - This is a common mistake. The candidate focuses too much on providing the appropriate treatment and forgets to clear the patient prior to defibrillating.
   - Not only must you state "clear," you must visually look at the entire patient to ensure nobody is in contact.

4. **Inability to deliver DC (direct current) shock [does not use machine properly].**
   - You must ensure familiarity with all of the functions of the monitor/defibrillator at the station.
   - If you are not familiar with the type of machine at the station, the examiner will take a few moments to familiarize you with the basic functions of the equipment.

5. **Failure to demonstrate acceptable shock sequence.**
   - Initially, deliver *one* shock with 360 J monophasic (or biphasic equivalent) and *immediately* initiate/resume CPR, beginning with chest compressions.
   - Defibrillate *one* time, if indicated, after every 2 minutes of CPR.
   - After *any* defibrillation, immediately resume CPR.

6. **Failure to immediately order initiation or resumption of CPR when appropriate.**
   - The ONLY time that CPR should not be occurring is when you are defibrillating or assessing for a pulse.
   - There should be continuous activity during this station, just like in the field. If it seems like you are missing something, it is usually CPR. Remember, the examiner will not assume that CPR is ongoing unless you verbalize it.

7. **Failure to order correct management of the airway [ET when appropriate].**
   - Intubation should be ordered after the rhythm has been analyzed and managed appropriately and CPR is resumed.

8. **Failure to order administration of appropriate oxygen at appropriate time.**
   - If the scenario presents with a conscious patient, immediately order 100% supplemental oxygen via a nonrebreathing mask.
   - If the patient is intubated, be sure to verbalize that you have attached 100% oxygen and reservoir to the BVM device and have confirmed correct tube placement.

9. **Failure to diagnose or treat two or more rhythms correctly.**
   - You can see virtually any rhythm during this station; therefore, you must ensure familiarity with all of the basic dysrhythmias and their treatment, especially the following:
     - Ventricular tachycardia and fibrillation
     - Normal sinus rhythm
     - Sinus bradycardia and tachycardia
     - Supraventricular tachycardia
     - Asystole
   - Review the current ACLS guidelines and algorithms with regards to the appropriate management for the following rhythms/conditions:
     - PEA and asystole
     - Ventricular fibrillation/pulseless ventricular tachycardia
     - Wide complex tachycardia (ie, ventricular tachycardia with a pulse)
     - Narrow complex tachycardia (ie, supraventricular tachycardia)
     - Sinus bradycardia and the AV blocks

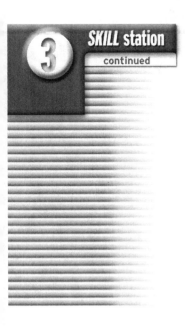

10. Orders administration of an inappropriate drug or lethal dosage.

- If you are unsure as to the correct dosage of a particular drug and/or what drug is indicated for a particular rhythm or condition, DO NOT GUESS! Continue with CPR and other therapies that you know are indicated (ie, defibrillation, correction of underlying causes of the rhythm or condition, etc).
- The more you review the ACLS guidelines and algorithms, the more familiar you will be with the appropriate drugs and dosages.

11. Failure to correctly diagnose or adequately treat ventricular fibrillation, ventricular tachycardia, or asystole.

- Again, be intimately familiar with the ACLS guidelines and algorithms to ensure that you know how to recognize and manage these deadly three rhythms.

Dynamic Cardiology Preparatory Questions

The ability to thoroughly and correctly verbalize all treatments, such as airway management and the management for all arrhythmias and/or conditions encountered in this station, is critical. Thoroughly writing out or even verbalizing the answers to the following questions will be an excellent way for you to practice.

1. List the components of the primary ABCD survey.

2. List the components of the secondary ABCD survey.

3. Describe your management of a patient who converts from ventricular fibrillation to sinus bradycardia **without a pulse** following defibrillation.

4. List, in the correct sequence, the appropriate steps of defibrillating a patient.

5. State the indications and correct **adult** dosages for the following medications in a **cardiac** situation:
   - Epinephrine 1:10,000
   - Vasopressin
   - Amiodarone
   - Lidocaine
   - Atropine sulfate

6. Describe the appropriate management for a status post cardiac arrest patient with a perfusing sinus tachycardia and a systolic blood pressure of 60/40 mm Hg.

7. Describe the steps to take **after** the placement of an endotracheal tube in an adult.

8. Describe the appropriate management for a patient with a narrow complex tachycardia at a rate of 180 beats/min, who presents without hemodynamic compromise.

9. What should you do after administering a medication to a cardiac arrest patient but prior to defibrillating?

10. How would you manage a patient in ventricular tachycardia **with a pulse**, who is hemodynamically stable?

Skill 3B: Static Cardiology

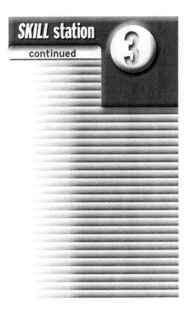

Station Time Limit: 6 minutes to complete all four patient scenarios.

Skill Station Objective: This skill is designed to evaluate your ability to recognize and verbally treat cardiac arrhythmias in accordance with current American Heart Association guidelines and algorithms. Four separate static ECG recordings with associated patient information will be presented. You may read the information aloud or to yourself. You will first need to verbally inform the examiner of your interpretation of the rhythm or condition, and then verbally inform the examiner of all of your treatments and interventions you would provide for the patient in the field. Assume that each rhythm you see in the 6-second strip continues in each patient and does not change. You may pass on any card and come back to it if time permits.

Your Partner(s): There are no partners needed for this station.

Skill Examiner Function(s): The skills examiner will present you with each of the four patient scenarios, record your actions, and monitor your time limit. The examiner is not permitted to provide any additional information other than what is presented within the scenario.

There are no predefined critical criteria for the static cardiology station. You must meet a minimum overall point value to successfully complete the station.

You must be intimately familiar with all of the basic cardiac arrhythmias and current ACLS guidelines/algorithms and be able to verbalize them accordingly. You are allowed a very short period of time to interpret the rhythm and verbalize the correct management for each of the four scenarios.

Static Cardiology Practice Scenarios

Presented here are four practice static cardiology scenarios. Read the scenario, interpret the cardiac rhythm, and then list the correct management for each case.

Table 3-5

Static Cardiology Performance Checklist

Static Cardiology		
STRIP #1 Diagnosis: Treatment:	1 2	
STRIP #2 Diagnosis: Treatment:	1 2	
STRIP #3 Diagnosis: Treatment:	1 2	
STRIP #4 Diagnosis: Treatment:	1 2	
Modeled from the NREMT Performance Skill Sheet	**12**	

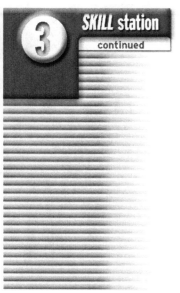

3 **SKILL station**
continued

━━━ Practice Scenario 1 ━━━

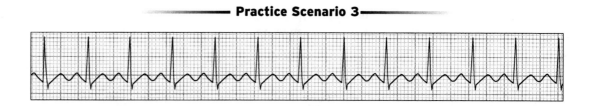

The patient with the above rhythm is a 49-year-old man who reports crushing, substernal chest pain and difficulty breathing. His blood pressure is 96/60 mm Hg and his respirations are 24 breaths/min and labored. His skin is ashen and diaphoretic.

1. Identify this cardiac rhythm/condition.

2. List the appropriate management for the patient.

━━━ Practice Scenario 2 ━━━

A 55-year-old woman with the above rhythm has generalized weakness, shortness of breath, and nausea. She has a blood pressure of 88/66 mm Hg, a pulse rate that corresponds with the ECG rhythm, and respirations of 24 breaths/min and slightly shallow.

1. Identify this cardiac rhythm/condition.

2. List the appropriate management for the patient.

━━━ Practice Scenario 3 ━━━

Your assessment of the 39-year-old man with the above rhythm reveals pulselessness and apnea. He has evidently had severe nausea, vomiting, and diarrhea for the past week.

1. Identify this cardiac rhythm/condition.

2. List the appropriate management for the patient.

━━━ Practice Scenario 4 ━━━

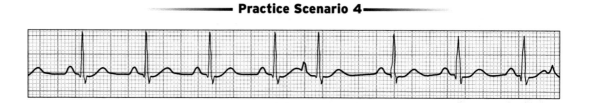

A 66-year-old man with an extensive cardiac history reports the sudden onset of crushing, substernal chest pain that radiates to his left jaw. He has a blood pressure of 140/92 mm Hg, a pulse rate that corresponds with the ECG rhythm, and respirations of 22 breaths/min with adequate air exchange.

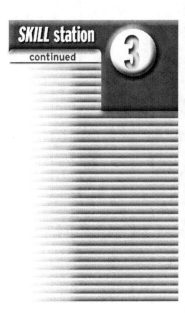

1. Identify this cardiac rhythm/condition.

2. List the appropriate management for the patient.

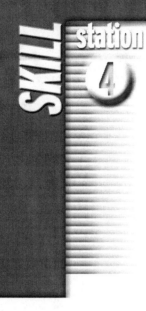

Skill Station 4: Oral Station**

Station Time Limit: 15 minutes for *each* of the oral stations (A and B).

Skill Station Objective: For each oral station scenario, you must verbally complete a simulated out-of-hospital patient encounter. You are responsible for all aspects of scene management and patient care for a given case. Since you cannot see the patient, you must verbalize *every* action, to include all interventions, questions that you would ask the patient, and any orders that you would normally give in the field. Throughout the case, you may assume that medical control has granted permission for you to perform any interventions that you request. You will also be required to complete a simulated radio report of this call just like you would in the field. You will be provided paper and a pen/pencil to take notes with during the station but must leave all materials in the room on completion of the station.

Your Partner(s): The make-up of your crew will be explained as part of the background information that you will read to the examiner at the beginning of this station. You are solely responsible for the actions of your partners. They will not do anything without your direction.

Skill Examiner Function(s): In addition to recording your actions and keeping track of the time, the skill examiner will play the role of the patient, family, bystanders, and other health care providers. Additionally, he/she will act as the receiving facility when you give your simulated radio report.

** Each candidate must complete two oral stations (A and B).

Table 3-6

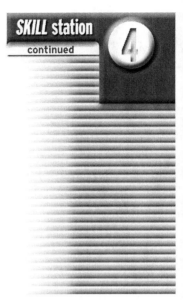

SKILL station
continued
4

Oral Station Performance Checklist

Oral Station		
Scene Management		
Thoroughly assessed and took deliberate actions to control the scene	3	
Assessed the scene, identified potential hazards, did not put anyone in danger	2	
Incompletely assessed or managed the scene	1	
Did not assess or manage the scene	0	
Patient Assessment		
Completed an organized assessment and integrated findings to expand further assessment	3	
Completed initial, focused, and ongoing assessments	2	
Performed an incomplete or disorganized assessment	1	
Did not complete an initial assessment	0	
Patient Management		
Managed all aspects of the patient's condition and anticipated further needs	3	
Appropriately managed the patient's presenting condition	2	
Performed an incomplete or disorganized management	1	
Did not manage life-threatening conditions	0	
Interpersonal Relations		
Established rapport and interacted in an organized, therapeutic manner	3	
Interacted and responded appropriately with patient, crew, and bystanders	2	
Used inappropriate communication techniques	1	
Demonstrated intolerance for patient, bystanders, and crew	0	
Integration (verbal report, field impression, and transport decision)		
Stated correct field impression and pathophysiology basis, provided succinct and accurate verbal report including social/psychological concerns, and considered alternate transport destinations	3	
Stated correct field impression, provided succinct and accurate verbal report, and appropriately stated transport decision	2	
Stated correct field impression, provided inappropriate verbal report or transport decision	1	
Stated incorrect field impression or did not provide verbal report	0	
Modeled from the NREMT performance skill sheet	**15**	

This skill, unlike any of the others that you must complete, takes away all semblances of patient and equipment simulation, which will require you to verbalize, in literal detail, how you would assess and provide total management of a patient, based upon a given scenario.

The oral station objective is to assess your critical-thinking skills and your ability to verbalize and rationalize all actions that you take. If one can verbalize how they would manage a patient, without the benefit of an actual patient in front of them, then they would most likely be able to perform in a similar fashion when faced with a real life situation.

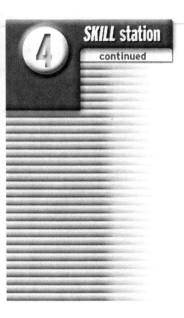

Critical Criteria: Oral Station

1.   Failure to appropriately address any of the scenario's "mandatory actions".
- For each scenario, there are actions or inactions that are specific to that particular scenario. For example;
  - A scenario involving a patient in insulin shock would require that you:
    - Obtain a dextostick and administer glucose.
    - Not administer the patient's prescribed insulin.
  - A patient with an acute asthma attack would require that you:
    - Administer a nebulized bronchodilator or subcutaneous epinephrine.
    - Not use any beta blocking medications.

2.   Performs or orders any harmful or dangerous action or intervention.
- This would be in addition to the mandatory actions specific to the scenario, such as not providing the appropriate oxygen therapy, administering an inappropriate or potentially lethal dosage of a medication, or performing a task that is clearly not indicated for the patient's condition and has the potential to cause harm.

Read the following sample scenario, to include the background and dispatch information at the beginning of the scenario and then the scenario's progression. This will give you a general idea of how you should approach this station.

——— Background & Dispatch Information ———

You are a paramedic functioning in a rural EMS system that responds to emergency calls only. Your partner is a paramedic as well. You are ten (10) minutes away from a minor emergency clinic and thirty (30) minutes away from a small community hospital.

At 1745 hours, you are dispatched to a residence for a patient that is "acting bizarre". It is in the middle of summer and the temperature is 100° F. Upon arrival at the scene, the patient's husband answers the door and directs you to the patient.

Table 3-7

Oral Station Scenario Template

Background Information	
EMS System description (including urban/rural setting)	Rural EMS system that responds to emergency calls only
Vehicle type/response capabilities	2 person paramedic level emergency medical service
Proximity to and level/type of facilities	10 minutes away from a minor emergency clinic 25 minutes away from the closest hospital
Dispatch Information	
Nature of the call	Patient is acting bizarre.
Location	Well kept walk-up single family dwelling
Dispatch time	1745 hours
Weather	100 degrees F, clear summer day
Personnel on scene	The patient's husband

Scene Survey Information

Scene considerations	No obstacles to the residence Stretcher access is only possible through the back door
Patient location	Large living room that is easy to maneuver a stretcher in
Visual appearance	Patient is sitting on couch, notably pale with beads of sweat on her forehead, the patient slowly looks up at you as you enter the room
Age, gender, weight	40 year old female, 120 pounds
Immediate surroundings (bystanders, family members present, etc.)	Clean, neat, well-kept surroundings Patient's husband is the only family member present

Patient Assessment

Chief complaint	Altered level of consciousness (acting bizarre per husband)
History of present illness/injury	The husband states "My wife just finished working in the garden outside. She came back in the house complaining of a headache. Shortly after that, she began acting bizarre. She ate one piece of toast about an hour ago".
Patient responses, symptoms, and pertinent negatives	Patient opens her eyes spontaneously but answers questions inappropriately

Past Medical History

Past medical history	Diabetes since childhood and migraine headaches
Medications and allergies	Humulin N 10 units SC AC breakfast, Humulin R 5 units SC AC breakfast, Midrin 2-4 capsules QD PRN
Social/family concerns	Patient lives with her husband, she functions independently

Examination Findings

Initial vital signs	B/P 94/60 P 128, rapid and weak R 24 with adequate air exchange
Respiratory	Lung sounds are clear and equal bilaterally
Cardiovascular	Tachycardia, slightly hypotensive
Gastrointestinal	Nausea
Genitourinary	—
Musculoskeletal	—
Neurologic	Opens her eyes spontaneously Confusion and hallucinations Pupils are midpoint and equally reactive
Integumentary	Skin is cool, clammy, and somewhat pale
Hematologic	—
Immunologic	—
Endocrine	Blood glucose 42 mg/dl
Psychiatric	—

SKILL station
continued
4

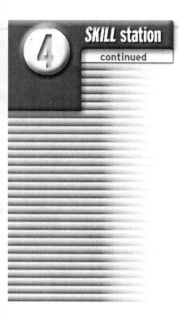

Patient Mangement

Initial stabilization	100% oxygen via non-rebreather mask
Treatments	100% oxygen, initiate IV, 25 grams 50% dextrose IV push
Monitoring	ECG – sinus tachycardia, SpO2 – 98%
Additional resources	—
Patient response to interventions	Patient is now more coherent and responds to questions appropriately

Transport Decision

Lifting and moving the patient	Place on ambulance stretcher
Mode	Prompt
Facilities	Emergency department

Conclusion

Field impression	Insulin shock (hypoglycemia)
Rationale for field impression	History of diabetes. Patient had breakfast, but then worked outside in the sun. Slight hypotension and tachycardia. Skin is cool and clammy
Related pathophysiology	"What is the basis for insulin shock in this case?" Strenuous exercise after eating a small meal
Verbal report	"Please provide me with a verbal report on this patient." Must include chief complaint, interventions, current patient condition, and ETA

Mandatory Actions

-Identification of potential life threats and prompt transport to emergency department
-High flow oxygen
-25 grams of 50% dextrose

Potentially Harmful/Dangerous Actions Ordered/Performed

-Administered patient's insulin to her

Modeled from the NREMT template for the oral station

You are required to ask a lot of questions in order to obtain the most information that will not only allow you to formulate a plausible field impression of the patient, but provide the most appropriate management as well. You are responsible for providing both a rationale and physiologic basis for your field impression.

Clearly, this is a station that requires a lot of forethought and literally staying one step ahead of yourself. The best suggestion is to verbally perform as though you were actually in the field taking care of the patient.

Unlike the patient assessment station, there is no skill sheet to practice with and clearly this skill is not as straightforward as patient assessment.

To best prepare for the oral station, you should choose a variety of illnesses and use the template above to review pertinent questions to ask as well as the most appropriate management for the illnesses that you choose. Remember; verbalize, verbalize, verbalize!

It is critical that you approach this station in the same manner in which you would approach an actual patient in the field. Let the patient's chief complaint guide your progression through the station. Not only must you ask questions specific to the patient's

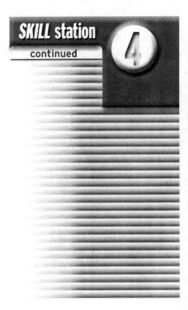

chief complaint (i.e. OPQRST, pertinent negatives, etc.), you must also inquire about medications, past medical history, and complete a review of systems, all of which could provide valuable information, thus allowing you to make a more plausible field impression or reinforcing the impression that you may have already formed.

You must voice all management that you would provide for the patient to include monitoring devices (i.e. pulse oximeter, dextrostick, cardiac monitor, etc.) and pay attention to the results of these tests. Reassessment of the patient after any interventions will assist you in making decisions regarding further management.

Just as you would in the field, you will have paper for documentation purposes. Write down all information pertinent to the patient. This will allow for a smooth verbal report, which you will be required to give. As mentioned on the performance checklist, the verbal report must be succinct and accurate. Consider using the following format:

- Your unit and provider level.
- Patient's age and sex.
- Chief complaint.
- History of present illness (i.e. OPQRST).
- Baseline vital signs.
- Pertinent past medical history, medications, and allergies (SAMPLE).
- Pertinent exam findings.
- Management provided and the patient's response (repeat vital signs).
- Estimated time of arrival.

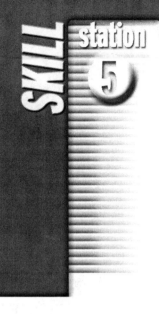
IV and Medication Skills

This is a combined station that will assess your ability to initiate a peripheral IV line and then administer a bolus of a medication given a particular scenario. For the purposes of this preparatory manual, we will break down the IV and medication stations into separate blocks so that you can focus on the criteria for each one individually. At the end of this section, you will be presented with three practice scenarios in which you will have to choose the correct medication, draw up the appropriate volume based on the concentration, and then properly administer the medication.

There are a variety of medications that will be available at this station and you will only be required to draw up and administer one. You should review the correct dosages of the more common medications (ie, atropine, epinephrine, etc) as well as your ability to calculate the appropriate dose in milliliters.

Note that in this combined station; if you are unsuccessful in initiating the IV line, you will not be able to administer the medication. Individual time limits and maximum number of attempts will be focused on for each component of this station.

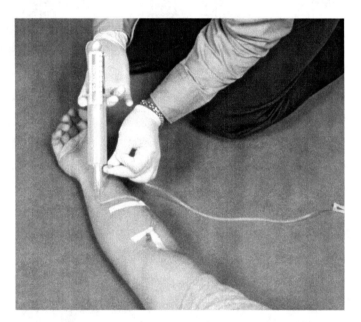

Skill 5A: Intravenous Therapy

Station Time Limit: 6-minute time limit to initiate and maintain a patent IV line.

Skill Station Objective: You will be given a patient scenario and will be required to establish an IV line just as you would in the field. You will have three attempts within the 6-minute time limit to initiate the IV. Although you are using a manikin arm, you should conduct yourself as if this were a real patient.

Your Partner(s): There are no partners required for this skill.

Skill Examiner Function(s): In addition to recording your actions and keeping track of the time, the skill examiner will play the role of the patient; therefore, you should ask him or her any questions that you would normally ask the patient in the field.

SKILL station continued **5**

Table 3-8

Intravenous Therapy Performance Checklist

Intravenous Therapy		
Checks selected IV fluid for: -Proper fluid (1 point) -Clarity (1 point)	2	
Selects appropriate catheter	1	
Selects proper administration set	1	
Connects IV tubing to the bag	1	
Prepares administration set [fills drip chamber and flushes tubing]	1	
Cuts or tears tape [at any time before venipuncture]	1	
Takes/verbalizes body substance isolation precautions [prior to venipuncture]	1	
Applies tourniquet	1	
Palpates suitable vein	1	
Cleanses site appropriately	1	
Performs venipuncture: -Inserts stylet (1 point) -Notes or verbalizes flashback (1 point) -Occludes vein proximal to catheter (1 point) -Removes stylet (1 point) -Connects IV tubing to catheter (1 point)	5	
Disposes/verbalizes disposal of needle in proper container	1	
Releases tourniquet	1	
Runs IV for a brief period to ensure patent line	1	
Secures catheter [tapes securely or verbalizes]	1	
Adjusts flow rate as appropriate	1	
Modeled from the NREMT performance skill sheet	**21**	

Critical Criteria: IV Therapy

1. Failure to establish a patent and properly adjusted IV within 6-minute time limit.

- Proper technique and taking your time will maximize your ability to successfully initiate the IV line.
- Try not to get discouraged should you be unable to initiate the IV on the first attempt. Simply explain to the examiner that you would remove the catheter and dispose of it properly, just like you would in the field.
- Use the following easy calculation formulae to determine how fast to run the IV:
  - KVO/TKO = 1 drop every 5 seconds.
  - 60 gtts/min = 1 drop every second.
  - 120 gtts/min = 2 drops every second.
  - 125 mL/hr = 125 gtts/min (based on 60 gtt/mL [microdrip] administration set).

2. Failure to take or verbalize body substance isolation precautions prior to performing venipuncture.

- Although the requirement is that you put on gloves prior to the actual venipuncture, you should play it safe and place gloves immediately or as mentioned earlier, wear gloves into the station.

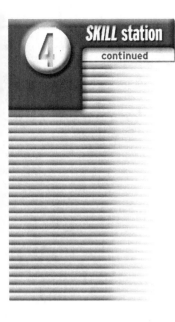

3. Contaminates equipment or site without appropriately correcting situation.

- The key phrase here is "without appropriately correcting situation." Just as it occurs in the field, we inadvertently contaminate IV catheters, the drip set, or the site after we have already cleaned it.
    - If you accidentally contaminate the catheter, dispose of it in the appropriate container and obtain another one.
    - If you inadvertently contaminate the proximal end of the administration set as you are attaching it to the IV bag, dispose of the contaminated equipment and obtain new supplies.
    - If you accidentally contaminate the venipuncture site, re-clean it appropriately.
- Mistakes are commonly made; however, not all are permanent. If you can *successfully recover* and stay within the 6-minute time limit, you are still meeting the standard.

4. Performs any improper technique resulting in the potential for uncontrolled hemorrhage, catheter shear, or air embolism.

- Here are some tips for preventing any action that would result in uncontrolled hemorrhage:
    - Use the preferred sites for IV initiation, such as the back of the hand or the anterior/posterior forearm first. As a last resort, use the antecubital fossa. Remember that the brachial artery is on the medial aspect of the upper arm so stay as midline as possible.
    - Should the examiner state that you have inadvertently cannulated an artery, you should state that you would *immediately* remove the catheter and apply firm direct pressure, followed by a pressure bandage.
    - After you obtain a flashback in the hub of the IV catheter, apply proximal pressure to the venipuncture site, loosen the tourniquet, and then attach the IV tubing. Make every attempt to avoid "bloodletting" as you remove the cap from the IV tubing for attachment to the hub of the catheter.
- Be sure that when you check the IV catheter for burs or other abnormalities, loosen the catheter on the needle. Do not slide the catheter over the tip of the needle as this could result in damage to the Teflon catheter, which would increase the risk of catheter shear.
- When you set up your IV bag and tubing, ensure that you completely flush (prime) the tubing prior to performing the venipuncture. A few little air bubbles are harmless; however, an entire line of air could easily cause an embolism.

5. Failure to successfully establish IV within three attempts during 6-minute time limit.

- Again, do not become frustrated if you are unable to successfully establish the IV on the first or second attempt. Regroup and approach it again. Just as it occurs in the field, all initial IV attempts are not successful.
- Many paramedics have "preferred" sites that they use initially when starting an IV in the field. For testing purposes, use the vein that you can most readily see, even if it is not your choice vein for field purposes. Whether it is on a live person or on an IV trainer, the best place to start an IV is where there is a "Y" (the juncture between two veins).

6. Failure to dispose/verbalize disposal of needle in proper container.

- The ONLY item that will be at this station that is red (other than blood) is the sharps disposal box. Be sure that you set it in a location where you cannot help but see it.
- To avoid the risk of forgetting to verbalize disposal of the sharps, physically place the contaminated sharps in the red box *immediately* after removing it from the catheter.

Skill 5B: IV Bolus Medications

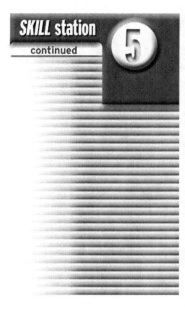

Station Time Limit: 3-minute time limit to begin the IV administration of a bolus medication.

Skill Station Objective: Provided that you were successful in initiating the IV line, you must choose the appropriate medication based on the brief scenario given, draw up the correct volume of the medication based on the concentration (mg/mL), and correctly administer the medication in a bolus (in one mass) form at the appropriate rate for that particular medication. Although you are using a manikin arm, you should conduct yourself as if this were a real patient.

Your Partner(s): There are no partners required for this skill.

Skill Examiner Function(s): In addition to recording your actions and keeping track of the time, the skill examiner will play the role of the patient; therefore, you should ask him or her any questions that you would normally ask the patient in the field.

Table 3-9

Intravenous Bolus Medications Performance Checklist

Intravenous Bolus Medications		
Asks patient for known allergies	1	
Selects correct medication	1	
Ensures correct concentration of drug	1	
Assembles prefilled syringe correctly and dispels air	1	
Continues body substance isolation precautions	1	
Cleanses injection site [Y-port or hub]	1	
Reaffirms medication	1	
Stops IV flow [pinches tubing or shuts off]	1	
Administers correct dose at proper push rate	1	
Disposes/verbalizes proper disposal of syringe and needle in proper container	1	
Flushes tubing [runs wide open for a brief period]	1	
Adjusts drip rate to TKO/KVO	1	
Verbalizes need to observe patient for desired effect/adverse side effects	1	
Modeled from the NREMT performance skill sheet	**13**	

After you have successfully initiated the IV line, you will immediately move to the IV bolus medication phase of the station. Note that for preparatory purposes, the performance checklist has been split between the two skills, when in actuality, both skills are on the same checklist. It is not critical that you verbalize BSI for the IV bolus medication station because you still have your gloves on from starting the IV.

Perhaps the most critical part of this skill is that there must be absolutely no doubt in your mind as to the correct medication to administer to the patient. You should approach this skill as in the field in that once you give a drug you cannot take it back!

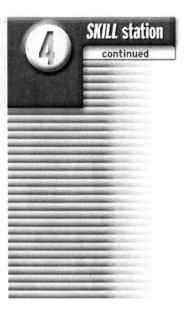

Critical Criteria: IV Bolus Medication Administration

1.   Failure to begin administration of medication within 3-minute time limit.

- Your time will begin as soon as the examiner reads you the brief scenario for the station. Be sure and pay attention to what the examiner is telling you. The scenario may outright tell you which medication to administer or you may have to choose the most appropriate medication based on the scenario and/or the patient's condition.
- The medication that is indicated may either be in the form of a prefilled syringe, which would only require you to state the correct volume of medication to give from the syringe, or you may have a multidose vial, in which you must physically draw up the appropriate volume. In either case, the examiner will ask to see the syringe to ensure that the appropriate volume has been drawn up.
- Be sure and review your ability to convert milligrams to milliliters. Some practice scenarios will be provided at the end of this section that will help you prepare.

2.   Contaminates equipment or site without appropriately correcting the situation.

- Remember that not all mistakes are permanent. If you take the appropriate steps to recover, just as you would in the field, and your time limit does not expire, then you have met the standard.
- Here are some examples of how the equipment or site might become contaminated and the corrective action that you should take:
  - You accidentally touch the injection port or top of the multidose vial after you have cleaned it.
    - Simply reclean the injection port or vial prior to administering the medication.
  - You accidentally touch the needle of the syringe or in any way contaminate the needle and/or syringe.
    - Discard the entire medication and obtain a new one. There should be ample amounts of medication in this station to allow you to do this.

3.   Failure to adequately dispel air resulting in potential for air embolism.

- Whether you are using a prefilled syringe or will have to draw up the medication from a multidose vial, you must ensure that all air is out of the syringe prior to administering the medication.
- Simply thumping the side of the syringe will force the bubbles to the top where they can be expelled prior to administration of the medication.
- If you must draw the medication from a multidose vial, draw approximately ½ to 1 mL more than what is required so that after you remove any bubbles, you can expel the excess air and still have the appropriate volume of the medication.
- The examiner may or may not ask to see the syringe prior to administration of the medication to ensure that there are no air bubbles. Assume that he/she will.

4.   Injects improper drug or dosage [wrong drug, incorrect amount, or pushes at inappropriate rate].

- Clearly, any of these mistakes could have grave consequences to your patient. You must review not only the medications that are indicated for particular situations, but the correct dosage, how the drug is supplied, and the appropriate rate of administration. You will be physically timed as to how fast you administer the medication.
- Here are some of the more common medications administered in the field, to include their indications, correct dosages, how they are supplied, the correct volume to draw up based on the dose, and the appropriate rate with which they should be administered. Note that these are based on adult dosages:

Medication	Indications	Correct Dose (IV or IO)	How Supplied	Appropriate Volume per Dose	Rate of Administration
Epinephrine 1:10,000	•Cardiac arrest ■ *Any* rhythm	1 mg (no max dose)	1 mg in 10 mL (0.1 mg/mL)	1 mg = 10 mL	Rapid IV push
Atropine sulfate	•Symptomatic bradycardia •Asystole •PEA (rate <60)	•0.5 mg for bradycardia •1mg for cardiac arrest	1 mg in 10 mL (0.1 mg/mL)	0.5 mg = 5 mL 1 mg = 10 mL	Rapid IV push
50% Dextrose	•Hypoglycemia	25 g of 50% solution	25 g in 50 mL (500 mg/mL)	12.5 g = 25 mL 25 g = 50 mL	Rapid IV push
Lidocaine	•Stable V-Tach •V-Fib and Pulseless V-Tach	1 to 1.5 mg/kg, then 0.5 to 0.75 mg/kg	Prefilled syringes containing 100 mg in 5 mL (20 mg/mL)	50 mg = 2.5 mL 100 mg = 5 mL	Rapid IV push

5. Failure to flush tubing after injecting medication.

• Do not forget to pinch the tubing proximal to the injection port prior to administering the medication. Doing this will not only allow a true bolus of the medication but will serve to remind you to flush the tubing afterwards. Run the IV wide open for approximately 20 to 30 seconds after administering the medication.

6. Recaps needle or failure to dispose/verbalize disposal of syringe and needle in proper container.

• The "never recaps needle" speaks for itself!

• The ONLY item that will be at this station that is red (other than blood) is the sharps disposal box. Be sure that you set it in a location where you cannot help but see it.

• To avoid the risk of forgetting to verbalize disposal of the sharps, physically place the contaminated sharps in the red box *immediately* after injecting the medication.

IV Bolus Medication Practice Scenarios

1. Medical control has ordered you to administer 5 mg of diazepam to a patient with acute anxiety. You have a 1 mL prefilled syringe that contains 20 mg of diazepam. How many milliliters will you give? What is the appropriate rate for administering this medication? Are there any special considerations for this particular medication?

2. A patient in refractory ventricular fibrillation requires 300 mg of amiodarone. You have medication vials containing 50 mg/mL of amiodarone. How many milliliters will you give? What is the appropriate rate for administering this medication? Are there any special considerations for this particular medication?

3. A patient with a heart rate of 40 beats/min and a blood pressure of 70/40 mm Hg requires 0.5 mg of atropine. You have a 10 mL prefilled syringe containing 1 mg of atropine. How many milliliters will you give? What is the appropriate rate for administering this medication? Are there any special considerations for this particular medication?

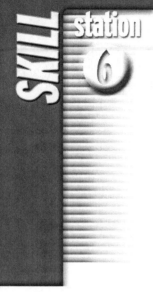

Pediatric Skills

The pediatric skills include ventilatory management of a child younger than 2 years and intraosseous infusion.

It is important to note that pediatric ventilatory management is not just a "small adult" station. You must select and use the equipment most suitable for the child's age (ie, an uncuffed tube, towels for maintaining optimum head placement, etc). Remember that the child's head is placed in a neutral or sniffing position as opposed to a more extended position used in the adult because of their proportionately larger head.

With regards to the pediatric intraosseous infusion, you should practice on a trainer designed for this skill. Many candidates practice on a chicken or turkey leg.

At the end of this section, you will be provided with two practice scenarios in which you must calculate, based on a child's weight, the appropriate adjusted flow rate for the intraosseous infusion.

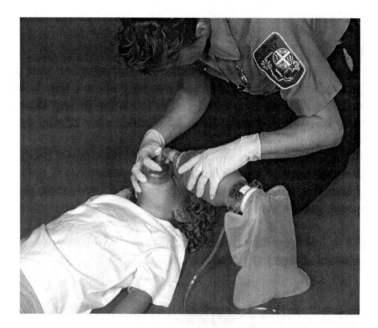

Skill 6A: Pediatric (younger than 2 years) Endotracheal Intubation

Station Time Limit: There is no set time limit for this station.

Skill Station Objective: This skill is designed to evaluate your ability to provide immediate and aggressive ventilatory assistance to an apneic infant with a pulse who has no injuries. This is a nontrauma situation, so cervical precautions are not necessary. You are required to demonstrate sequentially all procedures you would perform, from simple maneuvers and adjuncts to endotracheal intubation. You will have three attempts to successfully intubate the manikin. You must actually ventilate the manikin for at least 30 seconds with each adjunct and procedure used.

Your Partner(s): The skill examiner will serve as your trained assistant and will be interacting with you throughout this skill. He/she will correctly carry out your orders on your direction.

Skill Examiner Function(s): In addition to recording your actions, the skill examiner will serve as your trained assistant. You will be provided 2 minutes to check your equipment and prepare whatever you feel is necessary.

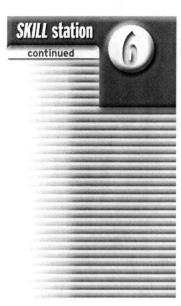

Table 3-10

Pediatric Endotracheal Intubation Performance Checklist

Pediatric (younger than 2 years) Endotracheal Intubation		
Takes or verbalizes body substance isolation precautions	1	
Opens the airway manually	1	
Elevates tongue, inserts simple adjunct [oropharyngeal or nasopharyngeal airway]	1	
Note: Examiner now informs candidate no gag reflex is present and patient accepts adjunct.		
Ventilates patient immediately with BVM device unattached to oxygen	1	
Ventilates patient with room air	1	
Note: Examiner now informs candidate that ventilation is being performed without difficulty and that pulse oximetry indicates the patient's blood oxygen saturation is 85%.		
Attaches oxygen reservoir to BVM device and connects to high-flow oxygen regulator [12 to 15 L/min]	1	
Ventilates patient at a rate of 12 to 20/min and ensures visible chest rise	1	
Note: After 30 seconds, examiner auscultates and reports breath sounds are present, equal bilaterally, and medical control has ordered intubation. The examiner must now take over ventilation.		
Directs assistant to pre-oxygenate patient	1	
Identifies/selects proper equipment for intubation	1	
Checks laryngoscope to ensure operational with bulb tight	1	
Note: Examiner to remove OPA and move out of the way when candidate is prepared to intubate.		
Places patient in neutral or sniffing position	1	
Inserts blade while displacing tongue	1	
Elevates mandible with laryngoscope	1	
Introduces ET tube and advances to proper depth	1	
Directs ventilation of patient	1	
Confirms proper placement by auscultation bilaterally over each lung and over epigastrium	1	
Note: Examiner to ask "If you had proper placement, what should you expect to hear?"		
Secures ET tube (may be verbalized)	1	
Modeled from the NREMT performance skill sheet	17	

As with the adult intubation station, this is not one of the more commonly failed skills. Intubation of a manikin, even though more difficult than on a real patient (humans do not have latex heads), is a relatively easy skill.

You must remember that as with all skills, lack of practice can turn what would have otherwise been simplistic into a frustrating event that will increase your anxiety and open you up for mistakes.

Be sure and practice with different types of pediatric intubation manikins. As with the adult, some manikins are easier to intubate than others and you will not know which one you will be testing with until you walk into the station.

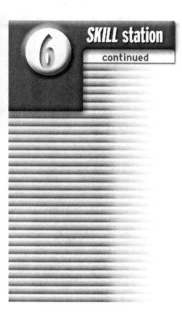

Critical Criteria: Pediatric Endotracheal Intubation

1. **Failure to initiate ventilations within 30 seconds after applying gloves or interrupts ventilations for greater than 30 seconds at any time.**
   - Remember, you have 2 minutes to prepare whatever equipment you think is necessary. It would be wise to fully assemble the BVM device if it is not already assembled. Also, get your oral airways in place so that they are easily accessible when you begin.
   - Thirty seconds may seem like a long time, but it can fly by if you are not keeping track of your time. There is no shame in counting out loud; 1 1,000, 2 1,000, 3 1,000, etc.

2. **Failure to take or verbalize body substance isolation precautions.**
   - As with all skills, if you walk into the station with gloves on, you are covered. Even though critical criteria #1 states that you must begin ventilations within 30 seconds after applying gloves, you still have 2 minutes to set up your equipment.

3. **Failure to pad under the torso to allow neutral head positioning or sniffing position.**
   - Don't forget to have a rolled towel sitting nearby. This will be provided at the station.
   - Remember that if you hyperextend a small child's head, the relatively large occiput will cause a reverse hyperflexion.

4. **Failure to voice and ultimately provide a high oxygen concentration [at least 85%].**
   - Initially in the station, you can either ventilate the patient with room air or begin ventilations with the BVM device already connected to 100% oxygen and the reservoir attached, provided that you do not interrupt ventilations for more than 30 seconds. In your setup time, it is suggested that you fully assemble the BVM device and have it prepared to deliver 100% oxygen. Just remember to verbally inform the examiner that the BVM device is attached to supplemental oxygen with the flowmeter set at 15 L/min.

5. **Failure to ventilate the patient at a rate of at least 12 to 20/min.**
   - Ensure that no matter what, you ventilate at least once every 3 to 5 seconds, which will ensure at least 12 to 20 ventilations per minute. Again, there is no shame in counting out loud. It beats having to repeat the station. The examiner will be timing you.

6. **Failure to provide adequate volumes per breath [maximum 2 errors/min are permissible].**
   - Remember that the most difficult part of using a BVM device with one person is to maintain an effective seal, especially if you have small hands. Practice using the c-clamp method to ensure that effective volume is delivered per breath. As long as the chest is rising well, you are providing effective ventilation.
   - Remember that with the small child, you must provide much less tidal volume than with the adult. Proper use of the pediatric BVM device will ensure this.

7. **Failure to pre-oxygenate patient prior to intubation.**
   - After you have provided a period of ventilation with 100% oxygen, the examiner then assumes the role of your partner. Remember to verbally inform them to pre-oxygenate the patient as you are assembling your intubation equipment.
   - Make sure that you had pre-assembled the BVM device to include the attachment of a reservoir and supplemental oxygen at 15 L/min. The examiner will NOT remind you of this.

8. **Failure to successfully intubate within three attempts.**
   - As previously mentioned, most candidates have trouble intubating because they are not used to practicing with the type of manikin that may be used at the test site. Practice with several different types.

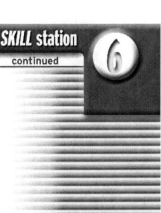

SKILL station
continued

- NEVER advance the ET tube until you have visualized the vocal cords. The best initial indicator of successful tube placement is when you visualize the tube passing in between the cords. A "blind" intubation will undoubtedly end up in the hypopharyngeal space (the esophagus).
- Don't forget to keep track of your time during your intubation attempt(s). You cannot interrupt ventilations for greater than 30 seconds at any time.

9.   Uses gums as a fulcrum.
- Using the proper technique with the laryngoscope easily prevents this. NEVER pry with the handle. Lift with the long axis of the handle instead.
- It takes very little effort to expose the vocal cords in a small child.

10.   Failure to ensure proper tube placement by auscultating bilaterally and over the epigastrium.
- The new AHA verbiage is "5-point auscultation." Have the stethoscope hanging around your neck as you are progressing through this station. This is a good prompt to remember to auscultate.

11.   Inserts any adjunct in a manner that is dangerous to the patient.
- Remember to correctly size the oral airway prior to placing it to ensure the most appropriate size. You must also demonstrate the correct placement procedure.
- Prelubricate both the ET tube and the mouth of the manikin to facilitate an easier intubation. You do not want to have to force the tube into place, which may give the examiner the impression that you are being too rough.
- Most importantly, know your equipment and when it is indicated.

12.   Attempts to use any equipment not appropriate for the pediatric patient.
- This is a child younger than 2 years. Cuffed tubes are NOT used.
- If you use a stylet (which you shouldn't), be extremely careful.
- Insert the tube to the appropriate depth. Use the following formula:
  - Depth of insertion = tube internal diameter (mm) × 3.
- Be sure and use the correct size tube. Remember these rules:
  - Use a tube the equivalent to the width of the child's small fingernail or,
  - Age in years / 4 + 4 = 4.5 mm tube for a 2-year-old child.
- A size 1 straight (Miller) blade is recommended for children between the ages of 1 and 2 years.

Skill 6B: Pediatric Intraosseous Infusion

Station Time Limit: 6-minute time limit.

Skill Station Objective: This skill tests your ability to establish an intraosseous infusion in a pediatric patient just as you would in the field. You will have a maximum of two attempts to establish a patent and flowing intraosseous infusion within the 6-minute time limit. Within this time limit, you will be required to adjust the flow rate to the proper setting based on the given scenario. Although you are using a manikin, you should conduct yourself as if this were a real patient.

Your Partner(s): There are no partners required for this skill.

Skill Examiner Function(s): In addition to recording your actions and keeping track of your time, the skill examiner will serve as the child's parent. You should ask him/her any questions that you would normally ask in this situation.

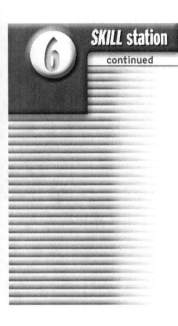

SKILL station
continued

Table 3-11

Pediatric Intraosseous Infusion Performance Checklist

Pediatric Intraosseous Infusion		
Checks selected IV fluid for: -Proper fluid (1 point) -Clarity (1 point)	2	
Selects appropriate equipment to include: -IO needle (1 point) -Syringe (1 point) -Saline (1 point) -Extension set (1 point)	4	
Selects proper administration set	1	
Connects administration set to bag	1	
Prepares administration set [fills drip chamber and flushes tubing]	1	
Prepares syringe and extension tubing	1	
Cuts or tears tape [at any time before IO puncture]	1	
Takes or verbalizes body substance isolation precautions [prior to IO puncture]	1	
Identifies proper anatomic site for IO puncture	1	
Cleanses site appropriately	1	
Performs IO puncture: -Stabilizes tibia (1 point) -Inserts needle at proper angle (1 point) -Advances needle with twisting motion until "pop" is felt (1 point) -Unscrews cap and removes stylet from needle (1 point)	4	
Disposes of needle in proper container	1	
Attaches administration set to IO needle (with or without 3-way)	1	
Slowly injects saline to assure proper placement of needle	1	
Adjusts flow rate as appropriate	1	
Secures needle with tape and supports with bulky dressing	1	
Modeled from the NREMT Performance Skill Sheet	23	

Correct technique, knowing your landmarks on the pediatric patient, and practice will lead to your success in this skill. The scenario that you will be presented with will either require you to give a fluid bolus, run a maintenance infusion, or both; therefore, revisiting your basic IV drip calculations would be a smart move.

Critical Criteria: Pediatric Intraosseous Infusion

1. **Failure to establish a patent and properly adjusted IO within 6-minute time limit.**
   - This time limit will allow you 1 chance per 3 minutes to complete the skill in its entirety. Don't rush; yet don't fly through it either, which would increase your chance of forgetting something.
   - If you are unsuccessful on the first attempt, take a deep breath, regroup and go at it again with the intent of being successful.
2. **Failure to take or verbalize body substance isolation precautions prior to performing IO puncture.**
   - Even though you do not have to put on gloves until right before you perform the actual IO puncture, take no chances of forgetting. Enter the station with gloves on.

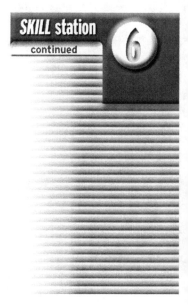

3. **Contaminates equipment or site without appropriately correcting situation.**
   - Again, the key phrase here is "without appropriately correcting situation." Just as it occurs in the field, we inadvertently contaminate IO catheters, the drip set, or the site after we have already cleaned it.
     - If you accidentally contaminate the IO catheter, dispose of it in the appropriate container and obtain another one.
     - If you inadvertently contaminate the proximal end of the administration set as you are attaching it to the IV bag, dispose of the contaminated equipment and obtain new supplies.
     - If you accidentally contaminate the IO puncture site, re-clean it appropriately.
   - Mistakes are commonly made; however, not all are permanent. If you can *successfully recover* and stay within the 6-minute time limit, you are still meeting the standard.

4. **Performs any improper technique resulting in the potential for air embolism.**
   - When you set up your IV bag and tubing, ensure that you completely flush (prime) the tubing prior to performing the IO puncture. Thump as many of the air bubbles out of the IV line as possible. Small children cannot tolerate as much air in their veins as adults can.

5. **Failure to ensure correct needle placement.**
   - Correct placement is verified by attaching a 5 to 10 mL syringe to the IO catheter after removing the trochar (stylet) and aspirating for bone marrow and/or blood. Easy aspiration confirms proper placement.

6. **Failure to successfully establish IO infusion within two attempts during 6-minute time limit.**
   - Technique, technique, technique!
   - Take your time and get it on the first attempt.
   - Don't get frustrated.

7. **Performing IO puncture in an unacceptable manner [improper site, incorrect needle angle, etc].**
   - In children younger than 6 years, the appropriate landmark is two to three finger-breadths below the tibial tuberosity (the bony protuberance just below the knee) and then medial until you palpate the flat area of the proximal tibia.
   - When performing the puncture, hold the IO needle *perpendicular* to the puncture site and insert it with a twisting motion until you feel a "pop." Once you feel the pop, insert the needle no further.
   - To avoid inadvertent slipping of the needle from the site during the puncture, grasp underneath the leg (upper calf area) and pull the skin tight over the puncture site.

8. **Failure to dispose of needle in proper container.**
   - Place the contaminated sharps (trochar) in the red box, which should be in an easily accessible spot, *immediately* after removing it from the IO catheter.

9. **Orders or performs any dangerous or potentially harmful procedure.**
   - Remember the correct procedure for performing this skill.
   - Bleed all air out of the IV line.
   - Ensure that you administer the appropriate volume of fluid at the appropriate rate based on the scenario.

Intraosseous Infusion Practice Scenarios

1. A severely dehydrated child requires fluid replacement. You are unable to obtain IV access after 3 attempts. Your protocol calls for an IO bolus of 20 mL/kg for the patient, who weighs 20 lb. What is the total volume to be administered?

2. A 5-year-old child has a weak femoral pulse and an unobtainable blood pressure. You are ordered to administer 20 mL/kg of normal saline to the child, who weighs 35 lb. What is the total volume to be administered?

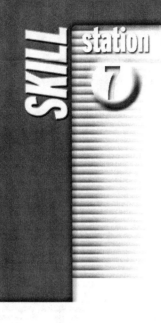

Random Basic Skills

This station will consist of performing one of three possible skills. You will not know which skill you will be expected to perform until you walk into the room. The three random basic skills include:

1. Spinal Immobilization (seated patient).

2. Spinal Immobilization (supine patient).

3. Bleeding Control/Shock Management.

You should put just as much practice into these basic skills as you do the paramedic level skills. The basic skills are failed more commonly than most of the advanced level skills because the candidate tends to focus less on them. It would be a shame to sail through all of the paramedic skills, only to get held up by failing the random basic skills. Unfortunately, this frequently occurs.

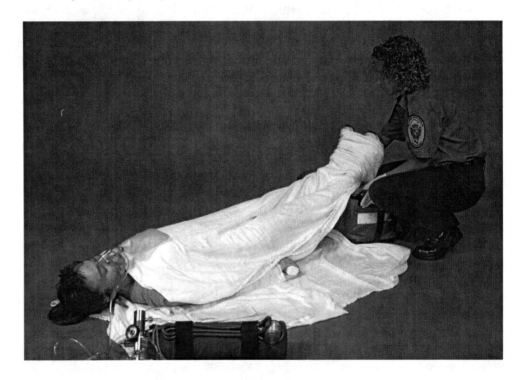

Skill 7A: Spinal Immobilization (seated patient)

Station Time Limit: 10 minutes.

Skill Station Objective: This skill is designed to evaluate your ability to provide spinal immobilization to a sitting patient using a half-spine immobilization device. You arrive on the scene of a motor vehicle accident with an EMT assistant. The scene is safe and there is only one patient. The EMT assistant has completed the scene size-up and the initial assessment of the patient; no critical condition requiring any intervention was found. The patient's vital signs remain stable. You are required to treat the specific, isolated problem of a suspected unstable spine using a half-spine immobilization device. You are responsible for the direction and subsequent actions of the EMT assistant. Transferring and immobilizing the patient to the long spine board may be verbalized.

Your Partner(s): You will have one EMT assistant who will perform any actions that you ask him/her to perform. The assistant will not perform any functions not directed by you.

Skill Examiner Function(s): The skill examiner will keep track of your time, record your actions, and check the effectiveness of immobilization on completion of the skill.

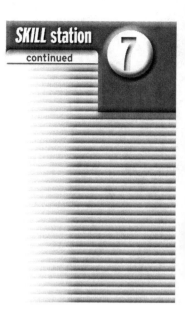

Table 3-12

Spinal Immobilization (seated patient) Performance Checklist

Spinal Immobilization- Seated Patient		
Takes or verbalizes body substance isolation precautions	1	
Directs assistant to place/maintain head in the neutral, in-line position	1	
Directs assistant to maintain manual immobilization of the head	1	
Assesses motor, sensory, and circulation function in each extremity	1	
Applies appropriately sized extrication collar	1	
Positions the immobilization device behind the patient	1	
Secures the device to the patient's torso	1	
Evaluates torso fixation and adjusts as necessary	1	
Evaluates and pads behind the patient's head as necessary	1	
Secures the patient's head to the device	1	
Verbalizes moving the patient to a long backboard	1	
Reassesses motor, sensory, and circulation function in each extremity	1	
Modeled from the NREMT Performance Skill Sheet	**12**	

Critical Criteria: Spinal Immobilization (seated patient)

1. Did not immediately direct or take manual immobilization of the head.
- ANY skill that involves trauma assessment or management is going to begin with you ensuring that the patient's head is in a neutral, in-line position. This skill is no different.
- Use your partner, as that is his/her intended purpose.

2. Did not properly apply appropriately sized cervical collar before ordering release of manual immobilization.
- Don't get this statement confused. Your partner must not release manual stabilization of the head until the patient is *fully* immobilized in the device.
- To ensure the most appropriately sized cervical collar, measure from the top of the patient's shoulder to just below the earlobe. A collar that is not the correct size will either cause flexion or extension of the patient's neck.

3. Released or ordered release of manual immobilization before it was maintained mechanically.
- To best avoid making this mistake, tell your partner to maintain manual stabilization of the patient's head and do not allow him/her to release it until after you have reassessed the patient's distal pulses and neuro status.
- There is nothing that says your partner must let go of the patient's head after the device is fully applied.
- Remember, the patient is not considered fully immobile until the entire device is applied.

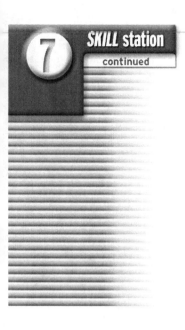

4. **Manipulated or moved patient excessively causing potential spinal compromise.**
   - Ensure that you inform your partner that no moves of the patient will take place without his/her command.
   - All moves of the patient, regardless of how slight, must be uniform, moving the patient as a unit at the command of the person maintaining stabilization of the patient's head.
   - Do not be too rough when applying the immobilization device.

5. **Head immobilized to the device *before* device sufficiently secured to torso.**
   - Securing the patient's head prior to the torso may cause unnecessary movement of the neck when the straps are applied and cinched to the torso.
   - Do not mechanically immobilize the head until immobilization of the torso is *complete.* Candidates will commonly position the device in its entirety and then go back and tighten the straps. This is a bad practice and should be avoided.

6. **Device moves excessively up, down, left, or right on the patient's torso.**
   - To ensure the most effective immobilization of the torso, when placing the device behind the patient, make sure that the device is snugly fit underneath the patient's arms.
   - After you have positioned but not secured the torso, step back, look at the patient to make sure that the device is centered, and then secure the straps.

7. **Head immobilization allows for excessive movement.**
   - Don't forget to use the most appropriately sized cervical collar.
   - Candidates think that the pad for the posterior of the patient's head must be used simply because it is in the case with the device. In reality, only a small percentage of patients (usually those with "hunchbacks") will require this. Most of the time, this pillow device is not needed.
   - To ensure effective immobilization of the patient's head, follow this recommended sequence:
     - Position the device behind the patient (snug fit under the arms).
     - When your partner calls for the move, move the patient as a unit until he/she is sitting *completely* back into the device. The spinal cord stops well before the waist; therefore, it is okay to flex the patient at the waist to ensure this.
     - Remember that it is the area between the lower back (lumbar) and the back of the patient's head that must be in an inline position at all times.

8. **Torso fixation inhibits chest rise, resulting in respiratory compromise.**
   - To ensure adequate, yet not asphyxiating security of the torso, ask the patient to take in a deep breath and hold it until you have secured the strap. Repeat this until all of the torso straps are secured. This will allow for adequate chest expansion within the secured torso.
   - Ask the patient if he/she is comfortable. If not, it is acceptable to loosen the torso straps and secure them as outlined above.

9. **On completion of immobilization, head is not in a neutral, in-line position.**
   - Remember, do not use the posterior padding device simply because it is there. Unnecessary use of this device is probably one of the most common reasons that candidates fail to effectively immobilize the head as it pushes the head forward.
   - Use the appropriately sized cervical collar as explained earlier.

10. **Did not reassess motor, sensory, and circulation functions in *each* extremity after voicing immobilization to the long backboard.**
    - Even though you are only required to assess motor, sensory, and circulation on completion of immobilization, get into the habit of checking it three times: initially, after the short device is placed, and then after verbalizing immobilization to the long backboard. The more you check it, the less chance of forgetting.

Skill 7B: Spinal Immobilization (supine patient)

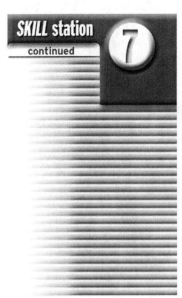

SKILL station
continued   7

Station Time Limit: 10 minutes.

Skill Station Objective: This skill is designed to evaluate your ability to provide spinal immobilization to a supine patient using a long spine immobilization device. You arrive on the scene with an EMT assistant. The EMT assistant has completed the scene size-up and the initial assessment of the patient; no critical condition requiring any intervention was found. The patient's vital signs remain stable. You are required to treat the specific, isolated problem of a suspected unstable spine using a long spine immobilization device. When moving the simulated patient to the device, you should use the help of the EMT assistant and the examiner (serving as a second EMT). The EMT assistant should control the head and cervical spine of the simulated patient while you and the examiner move the patient to the immobilization device. You are responsible for the direction and subsequent actions of the EMT assistant and the examiner.

Your Partner(s): You will have one EMT assistant who will perform any actions that you ask him/her to perform. The assistant will not perform any functions not directed by you. Additionally, the examiner will serve as a second EMT assistant for purposes of moving the patient.

Skill Examiner Function(s): In addition to serving as the second EMT assistant, the skill examiner will keep track of your time, record your actions, and check the effectiveness of immobilization on completion of the skill.

Table 3-13

Spinal Immobilization (supine patient) Performance Checklist

Spinal Immobilization—Supine Patient		
Takes or verbalizes body substance isolation precautions	1	
Directs assistant to place/maintain head in the neutral, in-line position	1	
Directs assistant to maintain manual immobilization of the head	1	
Assesses motor, sensory, and circulation function in each extremity	1	
Applies appropriately sized extrication collar	1	
Positions the immobilization device appropriately	1	
Directs movement of the patient onto the device without compromising the integrity of the spine	1	
Applies padding to the voids between the torso and the device as necessary	1	
Immobilizes the patient's torso to the device	1	
Evaluates and pads behind the patient's head as necessary	1	
Secures the patient's head to the device	1	
Secures the patient's legs to the device	1	
Secures the patient's arms to the device	1	
Reassesses motor, sensory, and circulation function in each extremity	1	
Modeled from the NREMT Performance Skill Sheet	**14**	

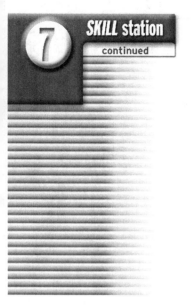

Critical Criteria: Spinal Immobilization (seated patient)

1. Did not immediately direct or take manual immobilization of the head.

- ANY skill that involves trauma assessment or management is going to begin with you ensuring that the patient's head is in a neutral, in-line position. This skill is no different.
- Use your partner, as that is his/her intended purpose.

2. Did not properly apply appropriately sized cervical collar before ordering release of manual immobilization.

- Don't get this statement confused. Your partner must not release manual stabilization of the head until the patient is *fully* immobilized in the device.
- To ensure the most appropriately sized cervical collar, measure from the top of the patient's shoulder to just below the earlobe. A collar that is not the correct size will either cause flexion or extension of the patient's neck.

3. Released or ordered release of manual immobilization before it was maintained mechanically.

- To best avoid making this mistake, tell your partner to maintain manual stabilization of the patient's head and do not allow him/her to release it until after you have completed the application of the cervical immobilization device (CID), which some people refer to as the "head chocks."
- Remember, the patient is not considered fully immobile until completely secured to the spine board with all straps placed and the CID is in place.

4. Manipulated or moved patient excessively causing potential spinal compromise.

- Ensure that you inform your partner that no moves of the patient will take place without his/her command.
- All moves of the patient, regardless of how slight, must be uniform, moving the patient as a unit at the command of the person maintaining stabilization of the patient's head.
- Should you have to move the spine board to place straps, ensure that this is done very carefully, without causing the patient to move on the board.

5. Head immobilized to the device *before* device sufficiently secured to torso.

- Securing the patient's head prior to the torso may cause unnecessary movement of the neck when the straps are applied to the torso and legs.
- Do not mechanically immobilize the head until immobilization of the torso is *complete*. Candidates will commonly position the device in its entirety, and then go back and tighten the straps. This is a bad practice and should be avoided.
- It makes no difference whether you immobilize the legs, torso, and head or the torso, legs, and head. *The critical element is that the torso is fully immobilized prior to immobilizing the head.*

6. Device moves excessively up, down, left, or right on the patient's torso.

- To ensure the most effective immobilization of the torso, when placing the patient on the spine board, ensure that he/she is completely centered. Remember, any moves of the patient must be uniform and at the command of the EMT assistant controlling the head.
- After you have positioned but not secured the torso, step back, look at the patient to make sure that the device is centered, and then secure the straps.

7. Head immobilization allows for excessive movement.

- Don't forget to use the most appropriately sized cervical collar.
- Ensure that the CID is properly positioned and secured appropriately. One strap should be under the chin of the cervical collar and the other strap should be over the patient's forehead.

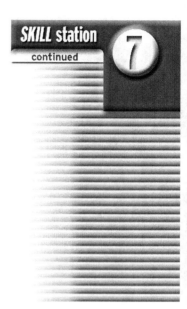

8. **On completion of immobilization, head is not in a neutral, in-line position.**
   - Use the appropriately sized cervical collar as explained earlier.
   - Make sure that when positioning the patient on the spine board, the patient is completely straight prior to immobilizing the head. Unnecessary moves to accomplish this only increase your chance of manipulating the spine.
9. **Did not reassess motor, sensory, and circulation functions in *each* extremity after voicing immobilization to the long backboard.**
   - Even though you are only required to assess motor, sensory, and circulation on completion of immobilization, get into the habit of checking it two times: before you place the cervical collar and then after the patient is fully immobilized to the long spine board.

Skill 7C: Bleeding Control/Shock Management

Station Time Limit: 10 minutes.

Skill Station Objective: This skill is designed to evaluate your ability to control hemorrhage. This is a scenario-based evaluation. As you progress through the scenario, you will be given various signs and symptoms appropriate for the simulated patient's condition. You will be required to manage the simulated patient based on these signs and symptoms.

Your Partner(s): There are no partners required for this skill.

Skill Examiner Function(s): The skill examiner will keep track of your time and record your actions as he/she provides you with the pertinent patient information.

Table 3-14

Bleeding Control/Shock Management Performance Checklist

Bleeding Control/Shock Management		
Takes or verbalizes body substance isolation precautions	1	
Applies direct pressure to the wound	1	
Elevates the extremity	1	
NOTE: The examiner must now inform the candidate that the wound continues to bleed.		
Applies an additional dressing to the wound	1	
NOTE: The examiner must now inform the candidate that the wound still continues to bleed. The second dressing does not control the bleeding.		
Locates and applies pressure to appropriate pressure point	1	
NOTE: The examiner must now inform the candidate that the bleeding is controlled.		
Bandages the wound	1	
NOTE: The examiner must now inform the candidate that the patient is exhibiting signs and symptoms of hypoperfusion.		
Properly positions the patient	1	
Administers a high concentration of oxygen	1	
Initiates steps to prevent heat loss from the patient	1	
Indicates the need for immediate transport	1	
Modeled from the NREMT Performance Skill Sheet	**10**	

SKILL station continued 7

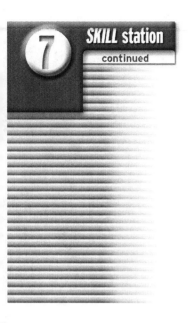

Critical Criteria: Bleeding Control/Shock Management

1.   Did not take or verbalize body substance isolation precautions.

- You have heard this for the last 11 skills. Do whatever you have to do to remember BSI, whether it involves wearing the gloves into the station or walking around all day with the gloves hanging out of your pocket so that you don't forget.

2.   Did not apply a high concentration of oxygen.

- Key in on the word "shock." All patients in shock receive 100% oxygen; however, do not negate prompt bleeding control for this.
- The scenario will start with the assumption that the airway is patent and the patient is breathing adequately.

3.   Applied a tourniquet before attempting other methods of bleeding control.

- At this point in your training, it should almost be second nature to slap your gloved hand and a dressing on a profound arterial hemorrhage and elevate the extremity at the same time.
- Think about it. How many people have *you* put a tourniquet on because you couldn't stop the bleeding by simpler means?

4.   Did not control hemorrhage in a timely manner.

- Prompt means immediately!

5.   Did not indicate a need for immediate transportation.

- This will be the last thing that you verbalize.
- Does it seem like you are forgetting to say something? Say transport!

Summary

Use the information presented in this section to your advantage. Focus on the steps and the critical criteria for each of the covered skills. Frequent practice of not only **what** you are doing, but **why**, will greatly enhance your overall performance. Remember that you must be able to be versatile, especially during the patient assessment and dynamic cardiology stations as the patient's condition frequently changes, requiring you to adjust your thought processes and management accordingly. The answers to the practice questions and scenarios in this section can be found in Section IV.

Answers and Rationales

Section 2: Practice Exam

Subtest 1: Airway and Breathing (30 items)

1. B. Although respirations at a rate of 18 breaths/min falls within the normal range for an adult, the presence of reduced tidal volume (shallow breathing) will result in an inadequate amount of oxygen breathed into the lungs.

2. C. Deeply unconscious patients, especially those who are intoxicated, are at high risk of regurgitation. The best device to protect the airway from aspiration is an endotracheal tube.

3. C. When breath sounds are not audible in the right hemithorax, especially following trauma, intrathoracic injury (ie, tension pneumothorax or hemothorax) should be suspected. Anatomically, it is nearly impossible to insert the endotracheal tube too far into the left mainstem bronchus.

4. C. To protect the airway from aspiration, the distal cuff must be inflated with 5 to 10 mL of air immediately following placement of the endotracheal tube. Inflating the cuff will also allow for a more reliable assessment of breath sounds because air will not regurgitate from the trachea and into the esophagus and vice versa.

5. A. A patient who can speak only in minimal word sentences (also called two-word dyspnea) is breathing inadequately and must be managed with positive pressure ventilations and 100% oxygen.

6. B. Because of decreasing peripheral perfusion with age, distal capillary refill is not a reliable indicator of an adult's ventilatory status. However, it is quite accurate in children younger than age 6 years. Remember that factors such as cold temperatures can affect capillary refill time.

7. B. To effectively manage a patient's airway, you must ensure that it is open and clear of foreign bodies or fluid. The presence of gurgling is an indication that the airway contains secretions; therefore, the patient must be suctioned prior to any further interventions.

8. B. Snoring respirations indicate partial airway obstruction by the tongue. The quickest way to remedy this is to perform a head tilt-chin lift maneuver, or jaw-thrust maneuver if trauma is suspected. After performing this maneuver, an airway adjunct should be inserted to assist in maintaining airway patency.

9. C. A severe airway obstruction is characterized by an inability to speak, extreme anxiety, decreased level of consciousness (ie, confusion, lethargy), falling oxygen saturation, and minimal or absent air movement. If the patient is coughing, it is weak and ineffective.

10. C. Signs of adequate breathing include, among others, bilateral chest wall movement, adequate depth (tidal volume), and pink skin (including mucous membranes). Tachypnea (rapid breathing) and hypopnea (shallow breathing [reduced tidal volume]) will result in inadequate minute volume.

11. B. The fact that the patient is easily able to speak would indicate that she is breathing adequately; however, the finding of perioral cyanosis indicates hypoxia. Therefore, supplemental oxygen should be given through a nonrebreathing mask at 15 L/min.

12. D. A respiratory rate of 32 breaths/min and shallow would result in an increase in the amount of dead space air. As the respirations become faster and more shallow, less volume reaches the lungs (alveolar air); therefore, it lingers in the area of the mainstem bronchus (dead space) and does not participate in pulmonary gas exchange. Both the tidal volume and minute volume would decrease.

13. A. Alveolar minute volume is the volume of air that reaches the alveoli and participates in pulmonary gas exchange. It is computed by multiplying the patient's tidal volume—less dead space volume—and the patient's respiratory rate. Dead space volume—the volume of air that lingers in the upper airway and does not reach the alveoli—is approximately 30% of the patient's tidal volume. Thus, if the patient's tidal volume is 450 mL, the *actual* volume of air that enters the lungs is approximately 315 mL (450 mL − 135 mL [30% of 450 mL] ÷ 315 mL). Therefore, the patient's alveolar minute volume is approximately 8,200 mL (315 mL × 26 breaths/min = 8,190 mL).

14. B. The first step that should be taken when you note minimal or no rise of the chest with artificial ventilation is to reposition the head to ensure that the tongue is not blocking the airway. If this is ineffective, other measures will have to be taken (ie, suction, intubation, etc).

15. C. Signs of inadequate assisted ventilation include minimal rise of the chest, significant air leakage from around the mask, an increase in the patient's heart rate, cyanosis that is not resolving, a falling oxygen saturation, and decreased ventilation compliance (increased resistance when ventilating).

16. D. Because no single method of confirming proper ET tube placement is infallible, multiple techniques of confirmation should be used. Regardless of the adjunct device used (eg, capnography/capnometry, esophageal detector device), it must be used in conjunction with *a careful* clinical assessment of the patient—auscultation of the lungs and epigastrium, observing for equal and adequate chest rise, and noting ventilation compliance. Because poor pulmonary perfusion results in decreased CO_2 elimination, the $ETCO_2$ detector is less reliable in such cases. Furthermore, elimination and detection of CO_2 following endotracheally-administered drugs—most notably epinephrine—can be drastically reduced.

17. D. Patients with a mild airway obstruction (eg, effective cough, adequate mental status, normal oxygen saturation) are able to move enough air to maintain adequate oxygenation. Leave these patients alone! Closely monitor the patient, encourage him or her to continue to cough, and transport to the hospital. Efforts to treat a mild airway obstruction with subdiaphragmatic (abdominal) thrusts may convert a mild airway obstruction to a severe one. Obviously, laryngoscopy is contraindicated in any conscious patient.

18. B. Because the rescuer is breathing air from his/her own lungs into the patient's lungs and both of his/her hands are freed to maintain an effective mask-to-face seal, the pocket face mask can deliver the greatest amount of ventilatory volume. A BVM device cannot deliver greater ventilatory volumes than a pocket face mask because of the difficulty in maintaining an effective mask-to-face seal that is often encountered.

19. C. During your 5-point auscultation following intubation, there should be NO sounds audible over the epigastrium, even if you can hear sounds over the lung fields. If epigastric sounds are heard, you must assume that you have inadvertently intubated the hypopharyngeal space (esophagus) and extubate the patient at once. A 2- to 3-minute period of hyperoxygenation must occur prior to further intubation attempts.

20. C. When a previously breathing patient becomes apneic, the rescuer must initiate two positive pressure ventilations (via either a BVM device or pocket face mask) and then assess for a carotid pulse.

21. A. The primary stimulus to breathe in a normal, healthy person is an increase in the level of arterial carbon dioxide. A decreased level of arterial oxygen is also a powerful stimulus to breathe but is not the primary mechanism in healthy individuals.

22. C. Because the patient is unconscious, an airway adjunct (oral or nasal airway) must be inserted to maintain airway patency. Since the rate of respirations is adequate (14 breaths/min with good chest rise), supplemental oxygen via a nonrebreathing mask should be applied. Continued monitoring for signs of inadequate breathing, which would require assisted ventilation and possibly intubation, is essential.

23. C. When ventilating a cardiac arrest patient after an advanced airway has been inserted (eg, ET tube, Combitube, LMA), do not attempt to synchronize compressions with ventilations. Perform 100 compressions/min and ventilations at a rate of 8 to 10 breaths/min. Deliver each ventilation over a period of 1 second—just enough to produce visible chest rise. Ventilating the cardiac arrest patient too forcefully or too rapidly increases the likelihood of gastric distention as well as increased intrathoracic pressure and decreased coronary blood flow.

24. C. In patients with severe COPD (ie, end-stage emphysema) and increased resistance to exhalation, you should attempt to prevent air trapping as this may cause inadvertent generation of intrinsic positive end-expiratory pressure (also called "auto-PEEP"). In hypovolemic patients—as with your severely dehydrated patient—auto-PEEP may significantly reduce cardiac output and blood pressure. Adjusting the ventilation rate to approximately 6 to 8 breaths/min—which will allow for complete exhalation—can prevent this. Manually-triggered ventilation devices (eg, demand valve) should not be used in any patient with pulmonary air trapping; use of such devices may result in widespread alveolar rupture and/or pneumothorax.

25. C. Although not nearly as common as with children, some adult patients cannot tolerate the oppressive feeling of an oxygen mask over their face. Should this occur, the paramedic should offer oxygen via a nasal cannula at a flow rate of 2 to 6 L/min.

26. D. In a patient who has sustained massive maxillofacial trauma and severe oral bleeding, intubation may be extremely difficult or impossible. Therefore, the paramedic may be required to perform an emergency needle or surgical cricothyroidotomy. Nasal intubation is contraindicated in the apneic patient. Because the mandible is used to maintain an effective mask-to-face seal, BVM device ventilations most likely would be ineffective when this structure is fractured. Digital intubation often takes too long and is frequently unsuccessful.

27. A. Prior to placing a nonrebreathing mask on a patient, you must ensure that the reservoir bag is completely filled. If it is not prefilled, the nonrebreathing mask will not deliver high concentrations of oxygen. The appropriate oxygen flow rate for a nonrebreathing mask is 12 to 15 L/min.

28. C. A room air oxygen saturation reading of 93% indicates mild hypoxia. Because the firefighter is awake, alert, and not showing outward signs of inadequate breathing, the initial airway management of choice should be to deliver 100% supplemental oxygen through a nonrebreathing mask at a flow rate of 15 L/min.

29. D. A markedly decreased level of consciousness and an oxygen saturation reading of 85% despite the use of supplemental oxygen indicate that this patient is no longer breathing adequately. Assisted ventilations with 100% oxygen should be initiated as you prepare for intubation to protect the airway before it closes.

30. B. A capnographer, also referred to as an end-tidal carbon dioxide detector, will tell you how much carbon dioxide is being eliminated from the body through exhalation. It is a device that is often used to provide secondary confirmation of successful intubation.

Subtest 2: Cardiology (30 items)

1. C. Chest pain of cardiac origin is most often described as crushing, dull, pressure, or as a feeling of heaviness. Bear in mind that these are typical pain descriptions. The paramedic should not rule out a cardiac problem if the patient describes the pain differently.

2. D. The rhythm shown is sinus tachycardia. Any increase in cardiac workload, such as an increased heart rate or blood pressure, will increase the amount of oxygen that the myocardium demands and consumes. This could extend the area of ischemic heart muscle and enlarge the area of an acute myocardial infarction.

3. B. Cephalgia, more commonly known as a headache, is not a common sign associated with cardiac compromise.

4. B. According to the American Heart Association, most cases of adult cardiac arrest are secondary to a cardiac arrhythmia, most frequently ventricular fibrillation. This underscores the criticality of early defibrillation.

5. B. Aspirin should be administered as soon as possible to any patient with signs and symptoms of acute coronary syndrome (eg, unstable angina, myocardial infarction). Aspirin blocks the formation of thromboxane A_2, thus minimizing local coronary vasoconstriction and making the platelets less "sticky." The other interventions listed in this question—IV therapy, nitroglycerin, 12-lead acquisition—are indicated for this patient; however, early administration of aspirin has clearly been shown to reduce mortality and morbidity in patients with acute coronary syndrome.

6. A. Because of the typical "sawtooth" or flutter (F) waves, this rhythm is interpreted as atrial flutter. The block is fixed in that the ratio of "F" waves to QRS complexes is consistent (2:1).

7. C. Unless associated with a fast rate (> 100 beats/min) and hemodynamic compromise (eg, hypotension, decreased mental status, pulmonary edema), treatment for atrial flutter simply involves close monitoring and prompt transport. The patient's chest pain is likely the result of acute coronary syndrome, not his cardiac rhythm. Therefore, cardioversion or pharmacologic treatment (eg, amiodarone, diltiazem) for his atrial flutter is not indicated at this point.

8. C. Secondary ventricular fibrillation (VF), which has a higher mortality rate than primary VF, is the result of a sudden, catastrophic event such as an acute myocardial infarction, massive pulmonary embolism, or a ruptured cerebral aneurysm. Primary VF, which represents the majority of cardiac arrest cases, is the result of a sudden cardiac arrhythmia, often times in an otherwise healthy person.

9. B. Because of the patient's history of chest pain for 48 hours and her unstable vital signs, she is most likely in cardiogenic shock. Prior to infusing a vasopressor such as dopamine, a 250 to 500 mL bolus of normal saline solution should be given to rule out any hypovolemic element to her hypotension. Drugs such as morphine or nitroglycerin may further decrease the patient's blood pressure.

10. C. Waking up in the middle of the night with severe difficulty breathing (paroxysmal nocturnal dyspnea, or PND) and the dried blood on the patient's lips (from coughing up pink, frothy sputum) are consistent with left-sided heart failure.

11. C. Your initial action when managing a patient with asystole is to rule out the possibility of fine ventricular fibrillation because the treatment differs significantly. This can be accomplished by either viewing another lead and/or increasing the gain sensitivity on the cardiac monitor.

12. B. Lidocaine is used to treat ventricular dysrhythmias (ie, V-Fib, V-Tach); it is contraindicated in patients with asystole. Epinephrine and atropine are both indicated in the treatment of asystole. A *one-time dose* of vasopressin (40 units) can be given to patients with asystole to replace the first or second dose of epinephrine.

13. A. Leads II, III, and aVF view the inferior myocardial wall. ST segment elevation that is ≥ 2-mm and is present in two or more contiguous leads is suggestive of myocardial injury. In contrast to myocardial injury, ischemia is characterized by ST segment depression and/or T wave inversion. Remember that a "normal" 12-lead ECG does *not* rule out a cardiac event.

14. D. This rhythm is regular, with a rate of approximately 40 to 50 beats/min. It has widened QRS complexes and more P waves than QRS complexes. Because there is absolutely no relationship between any one P wave to a given QRS complex, this is a third-degree AV block, also called complete heart block.

15. B. AEDs are *only* applied to patients who are pulseless and apneic. If you are caring for a patient who is at risk for cardiac arrest, the AED should be readily available, but not attached to the patient. When used in children between 1 and 8 years of age, a dose-attenuating system (energy reducer) should be used in conjunction with pediatric-sized defibrillation pads. However, if these are not available, a regular AED should be applied. AEDs have a high specificity for recognizing shockable cardiac rhythms (eg, V-fib, pulseless V-tach); this means that they are very reliable. If the AED senses patient movement, it will not analyze the cardiac rhythm; you will receive a "check patient" message.

16. D. Whenever there is a change in rhythm during resuscitation, either from good to bad or vice versa, the paramedic should immediately assess for the presence of a carotid pulse.

17. C. Nitroglycerin acts as a smooth muscle relaxant. When given to a patient with cardiac-related chest pain, it dilates the coronary arteries, which increases oxygen supply to the myocardium. It also results in systemic pooling of blood through vasodilation and decreases preload (the amount of blood returned to the right atrium). This effect decreases the workload of the myocardium.

18. A. The correct dosing regimen of adenosine for a narrow complex tachycardia is 6 mg by rapid IV push, followed by 12 mg, which may be repeated once for a total dose of 30 mg (6, 12, and 12). Because of its short half-life of approximately 10 to 15 seconds, the medication must be given over a period of 1 to 3 seconds followed by a rapid saline solution flush with the arm elevated.

19. D. This patient, who is most likely very physically fit, is hemodynamically stable with a pulse rate of 42 beats/min; therefore, no interventions are necessary unless serious signs and/or symptoms are noted such as chest pain, shortness of breath, a decreased mental state, or hypotension.

20. C. When questioning patients about any type of pain, the paramedic should use open-ended questions whenever possible. This allows the patient to describe the pain in his/her own words and does not allow them the choice of simply answering yes or no, which may not truly be reflective of what they are feeling.

21. D. Although acute myocardial infarction should be highly suspected in any patient with chest pain, angina pectoris classically occurs with exertion or whenever there is an increase in myocardial oxygen demand. Because the pain from an acute myocardial infarction represents complete or near complete coronary artery blockage, the pain typically begins even when the patient is not exerting himself (ie, when asleep). A normal electrocardiogram alone does not rule in or out an acute myocardial infarction.

22. C. If ventricular fibrillation develops after a patient has undergone synchronized cardioversion, the paramedic must first ensure that the monitor is not in synchronize mode prior to defibrillating. Since there are no R waves to synchronize with, the monitor will not defibrillate ventricular fibrillation if the synchronizer is on.

23. D. Because of the importance of defibrillation, any delay in establishing IV access or intubation should not delay this critical intervention. If V-fib persists, defibrillate the patient with 360 joules and immediately resume CPR. Avoid unnecessary interruptions in CPR; limit interruptions to 10 seconds or less.

24. C. The patient is in monomorphic ventricular tachycardia with a pulse. The diaphoresis and hypotension (80/60 mm Hg) indicate that he is hemodynamically unstable; therefore, the treatment of choice is cardioversion beginning at 100 joules.

25. C. Pulseless electrical activity (PEA) with a rate of less than 60 beats/min should be managed with CPR, securing an endotracheal tube or establishing IV access (whichever comes first), and then administering 1 mg of epinephrine every 3 to 5 minutes and 1 mg of atropine every 3 to 5 minutes. If the rate of the rhythm in PEA is greater than 60 beats/min, atropine is not indicated.

26. B. Hypovolemia is most likely one of the easiest problems to manage in the field. Fluid boluses are repeatedly given, followed by a reassessment of the patient's condition. Remember, myocardial contraction is dependent on electricity and pressure. This pressure is caused by blood coursing through the myocardium. If there is no blood, the heart will not pump, even though electrical activity continues.

27. D. Following resuscitation to a perfusing rhythm, as evidenced by the presence of a pulse, the paramedic should immediately reassess the patient's airway status and continue to treat accordingly.

28. B. First, convert the patient's weight from pounds to kilograms: 145 ÷ 2.2 = 66 kg. Next, determine the desired dose: 15 µg/kg/min × 66 kg = 990 µg/min. The next step is to determine the concentration of dopamine on hand: 800 mg ÷ 500 mL = 1.6 mg/mL (1,600 µg/mL [1.6 × 1,000 = 1,600]). Now, you must determine the number of mL to be delivered per minute: 990 µg/min [desired dose] ÷ 1,600 µg/mL [concentration on hand] = 0.6 mL/min. The final step is to determine the number of drops per minute that you must set your IV flow rate at: 0.6 mL/min × 60 gtts/mL (drip factor of the microdrip) ÷ 1 (total infusion time in minutes) = 36 gtts/min.

29. D. A major emphasis is placed on minimizing interruptions in CPR. Research has shown that even a brief pause in chest compressions can result in a significant decrease in coronary and cerebral perfusion. Therefore, CPR should be continuing—even as the defibrillator is charging. When the defibrillator is charged, ensure (visually and verbally) that nobody is touching the patient, and then deliver the shock. When defibrillating a patient with V-fib, you must ensure that the synchronizer is off; the synchronizer will not be able to identify an R wave in V-fib due to the chaotic nature of the dysrhythmia. Adult patients in cardiac arrest should be ventilated at a rate of 8 to 10 breaths/min. Excessive ventilation rates may lead to increased intrathoracic pressure, thus impeding venous return and cardiac output.

30. D. Because third-degree AV block (complete heart block)—an inherently slow cardiac dysrhythmia—represents total atrioventricular dissociation, it is associated with hemodynamic compromise in most cases and should be treated with immediate transcutaneous pacing (TCP). Signs of hemodynamic compromise include, among others, pulmonary edema, decreased level of consciousness, shortness of breath, and hypotension. First degree AV block is typically a benign rhythm and is uncommonly associated with bradycardia and hemodynamic instability. TCP is not indicated in patients with PEA, nor would it be effective in patients with prolonged asystole.

Subtest 3: Trauma (30 items)

1. B. Any problem with the airway poses an immediate threat to life. Examples include pneumothorax (open and closed), airway obstruction, and pulmonary edema. An open pneumothorax (sucking chest wound) must be sealed immediately on discovery. Bilateral femur fractures and a crushed pelvis frequently lead to severe internal bleeding, but airway problems always pose an immediate threat to life.

2. C. When securing a patient to either a long or a short backboard, you must secure the patient's torso prior to securing the head. If the head is secured first, it can be inadvertently manipulated as you secure the torso. Your partner must maintain constant manual stabilization of the patient's head until fully immobilized.

3. A. Slow, irregular respirations will not provide adequate minute volume and should be treated with ventilation assistance. Use a BVM device initially, until you are ready to definitively secure the patient's airway. After a 2- to 3-minute period of preoxygenation with a BVM, you should proceed with rapid sequence intubation (RSI), which involves administering a potent sedative-hypnotic drug (ie, Versed, Valium) and a neuromuscular blocking drug (ie, Norcuron, Zemuron). Because the patient is bleeding from the nose—a sign of closed head trauma—nasotracheal intubation is contraindicated. A nonrebreathing mask does not deliver oxygen via positive-pressure; therefore, it will be of little to no benefit in treating this patient's inadequate breathing.

4. D. Relative to the baseline vital signs, an increase in the blood pressure and a decrease in the pulse are most indicative of increased intracranial pressure. The trio of hypertension, bradycardia, and altered breathing is referred to as "Cushing's Triad" and is a classic finding in patients with increased intracranial pressure.

5. D. The most appropriate management for a patient with isolated head trauma and vital signs suggestive of such includes ventilatory assistance (if the breathing is inadequate), restriction of fluids to avoid further increases in intracranial pressure, and rapid transport to the hospital. Overzealous ventilation, which results in cerebral vasoconstriction, can cause or worsen cerebral hypoxia.

6. A. Flattened neck veins and unilaterally diminished or absent breath sounds that are dull to percussion suggest a hemothorax. If these findings are discovered in the rapid trauma assessment, you should initiate shock management and continue with the assessment. Needle thoracentesis is not indicated for a hemothorax.

7. B. A laceration to the femoral artery and hypertension would be the most difficult to control. This is because the femoral artery is very large and hypertension increases the force of blood through the artery, thus increasing the severity of the bleeding. As the blood pressure falls, arterial blood loses it driving force, thus making it easier to control.

8. C. Prior to providing care, you must ensure that you and the patient are in a place of safety. Once this is ensured, assessment and management of the patient can begin.

9. A. Using the adult Rule of Nines, the anterior trunk, which accounts for 18% of the body surface area, is divided into the thorax and the abdomen. Therefore, a burn to the anterior thorax (half of the trunk) would account for 9% of the body surface area.

10. D. A typical pattern of injury is seen when a patient falls and lands on the feet. As a result of axial loading, the patient frequently sustains injury to the calcaneus (heels) as the initial point of impact. The force then travels upwards, causing injury to the hips. The force can be severe enough to result in injury to the relatively unprotected lumbar spine.

11. A. A rapid extrication, which is indicated in patients who are unstable, is performed by applying an extrication collar and rotating the patient onto a long backboard for removal from the automobile. A vest-style device takes too much time to apply and use of a short backboard is not indicated for rapid extraction of the patient. If the patient or the paramedic's life is in imminent danger, the patient is literally grabbed and dragged from the car while providing as much protection of the spine as possible.

12. D. Proprioception is the ability to sense the position, location, orientation and movement of a part of the body in relation to another. Muscles, tendons, joints and the inner ear contain proprioceptors, which relay positional information to the brain. The brain then analyzes this information and provides us with a sense of body orientation and movement. The inability of a patient to comprehend questions is called receptive aphasia. A spinal injury usually results in a decrease or absence of sensory and motor functions distal to the injury site. The condition in which the body's temperature assumes that of the environment is called poikilothermia.

13. C. An open wound to the chest (sucking chest wound) must be sealed immediately on discovery so that air is not sucked into the wound, resulting in inadequate ventilation of the affected lung.

14. B. There are two indications for removing impaled objects: when they are impaled through the cheek and/or threaten the airway and when they interfere with your ability to perform CPR. Because chest compressions are performed in the precordial area, the knife must be removed in this patient.

15. C. Bleeding from the groin area indicates a femoral arterial bleed. The patient will exanguinate (bleed to death) if this bleeding is not controlled immediately. Once this has been accomplished, the patient must be removed from the car with the rapid extrication technique.

16. A. Bleeding or other fluid drainage from the nose following head trauma is indicative of a fracture of the cribriform plate. The cribriform plate is essentially the floor of the brain. When a fracture to this plate occurs, cerebrospinal fluid (CSF) will leak into the sinuses and drain from the nose. CSF drainage from the ears is indicative of a basilar skull fracture.

17. C. When assessing a painful deformity to the upper arm (humerus), the pulse most distal to the injury should be assessed (as with any orthopaedic injury). In this patient, this would be the radial artery.

18. D. Patients with a chest injury should have a cardiac monitor routinely applied to assess for and treat any associated arrhythmias. Use of a PASG is generally contraindicated for a patient who has injuries above the last rib. Bleeding into the chest cavity can be severe and may require fluid boluses and not a maintenance infusion. A needle thoracentesis is not routinely performed unless the patient is exhibiting signs and symptoms of a tension pneumothorax.

19. C. Significant mechanisms of injury include falls of greater than 20′ in the adult (or three times the patient's height), penetrating injuries to the head, chest, or abdomen, and the death of another person in the same car. Isolated impaled objects in the extremities generally are not considered significant mechanisms of injury unless there is severe bleeding.

20. B. A combination of direct pressure and elevation of an extremity is a common method of controlling severe bleeding from an extremity. Should this combination be successful in managing the bleeding, a pressure bandage should be applied. There is no such thing as a loose tourniquet.

21. D. Initial care for any soft-tissue injury includes controlling external bleeding. This is best accomplished by applying a sterile dressing to the wound. Assessing distal circulation can occur after the bleeding has been controlled. Irrigation of open wounds is not routinely performed in the field.

22. A. No airway, no patient! Prior to administering further care to a patient, airway patency and effective oxygenation and ventilation must be assured. Severe bleeding from the evisceration, if present, should be immediately controlled by the paramedic who is not managing the airway. Proper care for an abdominal evisceration involves covering the protruding bowel with a moist, sterile dressing and then covering the moist dressing with a dry one. Never replace the bowel back into the abdominal cavity; this significantly increases the risk of infection.

23. D. Signs of a pericardial tamponade include a narrowing pulse pressure (falling systolic and rising diastolic), muffled heart tones, and jugular venous distention. This trio of findings is known as "Beck's Triad." In addition, pulsus paradoxus, in which the blood pressure drops greater than 10 mm Hg during inhalation, may be observed in patients who have severe tamponade.

24. A. Hypotension and a normal or slow heart rate, especially with accompanying trauma to the spine, are indicative of neurogenic (spinal) shock. Because the sympathetic nerves originate from the thoracic spine, injury to this area will inhibit the release of adrenalin, which produces the typical tachycardia and diaphoresis seen in other types of shock (ie, hypovolemic, septic, etc).

25. C. Because full-thickness (third-degree) burns destroy all layers of the skin, the patient is prone to, among other things, hypothermia. Steps must be taken to prevent the loss of body heat in patients with full-thickness burns. Remember that the skin is a vital organ in maintaining body temperature.

26. B. Posturing, decorticate or decerebrate, indicates brain injury, usually in the region of the brain stem. Remember that the spinal cord must be intact for the extremities to move, either voluntarily or involuntarily. Priapism (sustained penile erection), paresthesia, and paralysis all indicate spinal injury.

27. C. Patients with isolated head trauma do not present with signs of shock; therefore, this patient probably has a hidden internal bleed. He must be managed with 100% supplemental oxygen and IV fluid boluses to maintain adequate perfusion.

28. B. Paradoxical chest wall movement is a classic indicator of a flail chest. Once this is discovered in the rapid assessment, immediate hand stabilization should be applied until the flail segment can be stabilized with a bulky dressing. Circumferentially taping the chest wall will impair breathing. It is important to note that even when an injury of this type is discovered, the rapid assessment should be continued following management of this finding.

29. **D.** One of the earliest signs of shock is tachypnea (increased respirations). Signs such as weak central pulses, absent peripheral pulses, and a rapid thready pulse all indicate a low cardiac output state and hypotension and are later findings in shock.

30. **B.** The patient with confusion would be the best candidate for a rapid extrication. Any altered mental status following trauma should be assumed to be the result of head injury, cerebral hypoxia, or both. Open head injury with exposed brain mater is an ominous finding that is generally not compatible with life.

Subtest 4: Medical (30 items)

1. **D.** The patient has signs of an opiate overdose (slow, shallow breathing, constricted pupils, bradycardia, and hypotension). The drug of choice would be IV administration of 0.4 to 2.0 mg of naloxone. Should this fail, atropine would be a consideration.

2. **C.** Central nervous system (CNS) depression, secondary to the effects of the narcotic that the patient has overdosed on, is causing the hypotension. Among other clinical signs, the bradycardia and the slow, shallow breathing are also the effects of CNS depression.

3. **D.** When a patient is in a situation that is causing harm or has the potential to cause harm (ie, extremes in temperature), the priority is to move the patient to a place of safety. In the case of a heat-related emergency, this involves moving the patient to a cooler area where the appropriate care can be rendered.

4. **B.** When glucose does not reach the cell where it can be used for energy, the cell will metabolize fat instead, which produces ketoacids. As the body attempts to rid itself of these acids, the respirations become deep (hyperpnea) and rapid (tachypnea), a phenomenon known as "Kussmaul respirations." Hyperglycemic ketoacidosis tends to manifest over several hours to even a few days. Because of the associated dehydration, the skin is generally warm and dry.

5. **C.** As evidenced by the signs and symptoms of anaphylactic shock, the patient requires 100% oxygen and IV administration of 0.3 to 0.5 mg of epinephrine 1:10,000. Administration of 25 to 50 mg of diphenhydramine hydrochloride is considered a second-line medication after epinephrine has been given. Subcutaneous epinephrine is indicated for mild to moderate allergic reactions.

6. **B.** Any patient with an altered mental status should be ruled out for hypoglycemia by obtaining a blood glucose reading. You must also keep in mind that a calm approach to the patient is important. The assumption of a psychiatric crisis is not in the best interest of the patient.

7. **A.** A persistent fever should alert the paramedic to the possibility of a communicable or infectious disease. HIV and tuberculosis both present with persistent fever of varying degrees. Diarrhea, sore throat, and a headache could indicate a variety of illnesses, not all of which may be communicable or infectious.

8. **C.** Since the patient is upstairs and removed from you, you and your partner are not in immediate danger; therefore, departing the scene is not necessary. However, you should remain in the ambulance until the police have arrived and secured the scene.

9. **B.** The worsening and persistent symptomatology that this patient is experiencing suggests a space-occupying intracranial lesion (ie, a tumor). Ruptured cerebral aneurysms and acute epidural bleeds present with a sudden onset of symptoms.

10. C. Your priority in the management of a possible overdose is to determine what was ingested. By identifying this, you can most appropriately manage the patient, which may include a specific antidote.

11. A. A burning sensation in the mouth or throat, headache, and a sympathetic discharge (hypertension and tachycardia) are indicative of cyanide poisoning. Management for this type of exposure includes having the patient breath amyl nitrite for 30 seconds, followed by 100% oxygen. Cyanide acts as a cellular asphyxiant, inhibiting oxygen uptake into the cell. This results in severe hypoxia, even in the presence of oxygen. The same burning chemicals that produce carbon monoxide produce cyanide. Cyanide poisoning can develop in patients who are on long-term sodium nitroprusside therapy.

12. B. Tinnitus (ringing in the ears), a craving for ice, and difficulty concentrating are all hallmark findings in a patient with chronic anemia. Other findings may include headache, dizziness, and tachycardia. Anemia is defined as a deficiency of red blood cells.

13. C. Factor VIII therapy is used in patients with hemophilia A. These patients lack that vital component of the blood clotting system. Administering medications such as aspirin or any others that thin the blood may result in worsening of any present bleeding, or may result in spontaneous bleeding.

14. B. The classic position for the patient with peritoneal inflammation or irritation is with the knees drawn up into the chest. This position takes much of the stress off of the abdominal muscles, thereby affording some relief.

15. A. It is contraindicated in the field to administer analgesia to patients who have abdominal pain. This will make the physician's evaluation of the patient difficult if the patient is pain free on arrival at the hospital.

16. C. Hot and dry or moist skin, deep breathing, and mental status changes are reflective of heatstroke. Contrary to popular belief, a patient can still have moist skin and be in heatstroke. A major differentiation between heat exhaustion and heatstroke is the patient's level of consciousness.

17. B. Patients with hypothyroidism have a very slow metabolic rate because of decreased amounts of thyroid hormone secretion. Any time the metabolic rate decreases, adequate heat is not generated; therefore, the patient is prone to hypothermia.

18. C. Prochlorperazine (Compazine) is an antiemetic medication that will not only relieve nausea from a migraine headache but has been found to be effective in terminating the headache itself. Patients with headaches such as migraines or cluster headaches generally prefer to lay flat (unless they are actively vomiting) with the lights dimmed.

19. A. A complex partial seizure, also referred to as a psychomotor or temporal lobe seizure, typically begins with an aura of varying degrees ranging from a metallic taste in the mouth to a "strange feeling." The patients are often confused and have difficulty with comprehension. Bouts of combativeness or even violent rage are occasionally seen.

20. D. A patient that has been having a seizure continuously for more than 5 to 10 minutes is said to be in status epilepticus. Once the appropriate airway management has been rendered, the next priority is to stop the seizure. Benzodiazepines, such as 5 to 10 mg of diazepam, are effective in terminating the seizure. If narcotic overdose or hypoglycemia is the cause of the seizure, naloxone and 50% dextrose can be given respectively.

21. B. Although the severely hypothermic patient usually does not respond to conventional ACLS therapies, one shock at 360 joules can be delivered if the patient is in V-fib or pulseless V-tach. If the patient does not respond to one shock, further defibrillation attempts should be deferred; the paramedic should focus on providing CPR and rewarming before reattempting defibrillation. If the patient's core body temperature is less than 86°F (30°C), cardioactive medications can accumulate to toxic levels if given repeatedly, and should therefore be withheld. Cardiac arrest patients with severe hypothermia should be intubated as soon as possible; doing so will protect the airway from aspiration and will facilitate effective ventilation with warm, humidified oxygen.

22. C. Though the mechanisms are different in salt water drownings as opposed to fresh water drownings, inadequate oxygenation and hypoxia are common in both and are typically secondary to laryngospasm.

23. B. Patients with blood glucose levels of 400 mg/dL and polyuria are dangerously close to hyperglycemic ketoacidosis, if not already there. High levels of blood glucose promote an osmotic diuretic effect, which explains the excessive urination. The result is severe dehydration. Field management is aimed at rehydrating the patient with isotonic crystalloid solutions. The patient definitely needs insulin; however, this is not a common field drug.

24. A. Signs of an allergic reaction include a fine, red rash or hives (urticaria), itching, and watery eyes. Once the histamine release becomes overwhelming, the cardiac and pulmonary systems are affected and the patient enters shock. Diaphoresis is a sign of shock; this is generally not seen in patients with mild to moderate allergic reactions who are not hypoperfused.

25. D. Rescue breathing, even when the patient is still in the water, will serve to immediately minimize hypoxia until the patient is out of the water and can be provided with more aggressive airway management that will most likely include frequent suctioning and perhaps even intubation. Prophylactic abdominal thrusts are not recommended because of the risk of regurgitation and subsequent aspiration of water.

26. B. Signs and symptoms suggestive of an extremely elevated metabolic rate, such as high fever [as high as 105°F to 106°F (40.5°C to 41.1°C)], hypertension, and profound tachycardia, especially in the patient with a history of Graves' disease (hyperthyroidism), are representative of thyrotoxic crisis (thyroid storm). This results from critically high levels of thyroid hormones.

27. D. Although the other treatments in this question would all be appropriate for a patient with thyroid storm (thyrotoxic crisis), definitive care includes rapidly transporting the patient to the hospital where medications can be given to lower the blood level of thyroid hormones, thyroxin being one of them.

28. B. This is a classic case of a black widow spider bite. The black widow spider typically can be found near wood piles or wood sheds. The patient will usually experience immediate sharp pain at the time of the bite, and then within a short period of time painful muscle spasms will develop in all of the major muscle groups. The black widow spider carries a neurotoxin in its venom, which explains the muscle spasms. If left untreated, CNS depression will continue and the patient's respirations and cardiovascular system will be affected.

29. B. Medications used to treat the symptoms of a black widow spider bite include 2.5 to 10 mg of diazepam or 0.1 to 0.2 mg/kg of calcium gluconate. These medications are used to relieve the painful muscle spasms caused by the neurotoxin in the spider's venom. Calcium chloride is not effective in the management of a black widow spider bite.

30. C. Insulin shock (hypoglycemia) is most noted for its rapid onset of symptoms, which includes loss of consciousness. Hyperglycemia, which leads to ketoacidosis, typically presents over an extended period of time. An ischemic stroke generally does not result in an immediate loss of consciousness like the hemorrhagic stroke.

Subtest 5: Obstetrics and Pediatrics (30 items)

1. B. The most effective means of controlling postpartum bleeding is to firmly massage the fundus (top) of the uterus, which results in constriction of the uterine vasculature. Another method is to allow the newborn to nurse as this will release the hormone oxytocin from the mother's brain, which also results in uterine vasoconstriction. Obviously, you should never pack anything into the vagina.

2. C. After providing two initial rescue breaths to an apneic child (1 year of age to the onset of puberty [12 to 14 years of age], you should assess for a pulse at the carotid or femoral artery. In infants (< 1 year of age), assess the pulse at the brachial artery.

3. C. In the initial assessment of the newborn, three parameters are assessed: respiratory effort, pulse rate, and skin color. The Apgar score is not a reliable indicator of the need for or extent of resuscitation since it is not assessed until the infant is 1 minute of age. Clearly, this is too long to wait before you begin your assessment.

4. A. Because a child's head is proportionately large in comparison to an adult, small children tend to land headfirst when they fall from a significant height as a result of gravity. This explains why falls with associated head trauma is the leading cause of traumatic death in the pediatric age group.

5. A. Expiratory grunting is an ominous finding in a child and suggests impending respiratory failure. It is the result of the child attempting to maintain oxygen reserve in the lungs.

6. C. The appropriate pediatric dose of epinephrine 1:10,000 when given via the IV or IO route is 0.1 mL/kg (0.01 mg/kg). Although the IV/IO routes are clearly preferred over endotracheal (ET) drug administration, the ET dose is 0.1 mg/kg (0.1 mL/kg) of a 1:1,000 solution. In certain situations (ie, beta blocker toxicity, status asthmaticus), higher doses of epinephrine may be required.

7. D. Multigravida describes a woman who has been pregnant more than two times. A woman who is nullipara has never been pregnant. Multipara describes a woman who has delivered more than one viable fetus. Primigravida describes a woman who is pregnant for the first time. Remember that gravida refers to the number of pregnancies and para refers to the number of live births. For example, a woman who is G3, P2 has been pregnant three times but has given birth to a living child only twice.

8. C. Luteinizing hormone (LH), which is released as the result of estrogen, is responsible for ovulation. Progesterone, along with estrogen, prepares the uterine lining (endometrium) for implantation by thickening its walls. Follicle-stimulating hormone (FSH) is responsible for producing estrogen. Human chorionic gonadotropin (HCG) prevents the corpus luteum, a yellow glandular structure, from degenerating so that the pregnancy can continue.

9. D. Pelvic inflammatory disease (PID) typically presents within 7 to 10 days after the end of the menstrual cycle and is characterized by bilateral lower abdominal quadrant pain, low-grade fever, painful intercourse (dyspareunia), and vaginal discharge. PID is frequently the result of a sexually transmitted disease such as chlamydia or gonorrhea.

10. C. A patient that has been sexually assaulted (male or female) should be considered a walking crime scene. Of course, management for any life-threatening problems has priority. The patient should be discouraged from changing clothes, bathing, or douching. Wounds should not be cleaned as potential evidence may be destroyed. It is preferable to have a paramedic of the same sex tend to the patient when possible.

11. C. Keeping in mind that the leading cause of nontraumatic cardiac arrest in infants and children is respiratory failure, aggressive airway management is critical. Signs of impending respiratory failure in a child include bradycardia, an altered mental status, and pale or cyanotic skin. If the child's pulse rate falls below 60 beats/min, chest compressions must be initiated

12. B. The most important initial question to ask after a child has had a seizure is whether or not there is a seizure history. This will allow you to adjust further questioning accordingly (ie, history of fever, recent head trauma, stiff neck, etc).

13. D. Seizure deaths are hypoxic deaths; therefore, your initial focus on a child who is actively seizing, especially one in status epilepticus, is to provide adequate ventilatory support. Once this has been addressed, measures aimed at stopping the seizure, which may include rectally administered diazepam, would be your next priority.

14. B. Current American Heart Association and American Academy of Pediatrics guidelines suggest that if a newborn has meconium present and is not showing signs of cardiorespiratory depression, free-flow oxygen should be administered as the assessment continues. If signs of compromise are present, such as poor muscle tone, apnea, or bradycardia, tracheal suctioning with an endotracheal tube is indicated.

15. A. Initial management for a nuchal cord (cord wrapped around the newborn's neck) is to gently attempt to slip the cord over the newborn's head. If this is unsuccessful, the cord should be clamped and cut.

16. C. According to the Brain Trauma Foundation (BTF), a child with a closed head injury and a Glasgow Coma Scale (GCS) score of less than 8 should be intubated. Clearly, the child's slow, irregular respirations require ventilation support. According to the BTF, the head-injured child should be ventilated at a rate of 20 breaths/min unless signs of brain herniation (eg, decerebrate posturing *or* no motor response to pain, fixed and dilated pupils *or* asymmetric pupils) are present. The efficacy of lidocaine in patients with head trauma is controversial; furthermore, the cited dose in this question—2 mg/kg—is too high for the child.

17. B. When estimating the lower limit systolic blood pressure for a child, use this formula: age (in years) $\times$ 2 + 70. Therefore, the lower limit systolic blood pressure for a 7-year-old child would be 80 to 85 mm Hg (7 [age in years] $\times$ 2 = 14 + 70 = 84). When estimating the upper limit systolic blood pressure for a child, use this formula: age (in years) $\times$ 2 + 90.

18. C. One of the most simplistic, yet effective ways of reducing oxygen demand in a child is to reduce anxiety (ie, omit unnecessary procedures, allow the parents to hold the child, etc). Another method is to maintain a normal ambient body temperature. If you make an attempt to increase the body temperature, the child's metabolic rate will increase, which requires more oxygen.

19. A. Management of third trimester bleeding includes taking measures to prevent shock (ie, 100% supplemental oxygen, providing warmth, etc). Volume expansion with crystalloids would be necessary if the patient were actually in shock. Uterine massage is indicated for postpartum bleeding.

20. C. Your index of suspicion for potential child abuse should increase when there is an unreasonable delay in seeking care for the child. This is not consistent care with that of a loving, prudent caregiver. Signs that a child is withdrawn or avoids contact with the parents would also suggest the possibility of abuse. Bruises to the tibias are a common injury pattern in small children, usually from bumping into furniture.

21. D. After tending to the child's injuries, you must remember that you are legally obligated to report any and all cases of suspected abuse. Accusing parents or care-givers of abuse will set you up for allegations of slander if you are wrong. When documenting the case (or any other case), you must only document the facts, not your opinion.

22. B. Signs of meningitis include, among others, fever, headache, and a stiff, painful neck (nuchal rigidity). A child who screams in pain every time he or she is picked up is doing so because of the traction that is placed on the inflamed spinal cord. This is called paradoxical irritability.

23. C. Signs of leukemia (cancer of the blood) include fatigue or weakness, easy bruising, and spontaneous bleeding. A patient with anemia can have similar signs/symptoms but tends to have cutaneous bleeding and an unusual craving for ice.

24. B. There is little in the way of emergency care that can be provided to a patient with anemia other than supportive care (ie, maintaining the ABCs). Definitive management can only be provided in the hospital.

25. C. Fever and fatigue are indicative of both HIV infection and tuberculosis. Kaposi's sarcoma (purple malignant skin lesions) is seen in HIV patients, as is *Pneumocystis carinii* (severe pneumonia). Hemoptysis (coughing up of blood) is a common finding in patients with tuberculosis.

26. A. As with any infection of the central nervous system, the patient is prone to seizures and must be closely monitored. It is recommended that you place a mask on the patient, not necessarily yourself.

27. C. When examining a patient who reports abdominal pain, you should palpate the painful area last. Doing so first will skew further evaluation of the abdomen because the patient will be in so much pain. This is especially true of children.

28. D. Provided that the child is not in shock (which he is not), your primary focus should be on transporting the patient where he can receive definitive care. A blood pressure of 90/50 mm Hg is considered normal for a child of this age. His other vital signs also are consistent with his age. Field analgesia should never be given to patients with abdominal pain. This will make the physician's examination difficult because the patient may be pain free on arrival in the emergency department.

29. D. Because newborns have immature immune systems and a decreased ability to produce pyrogens (fever-causing agents), fever is uncommon and suggests a significant illness, such as neonatal sepsis. Cooling is not recommended because of the risk of causing the newborn to shiver, which will only increase the body temperature and could precipitate a seizure.

30. B. A common complication in patients with tracheostomy tubes is obstruction of the tube by thick secretions. A child with bradycardia and an oxygen saturation level of 85% is showing signs of hypoxia. Prior to initiating positive pressure ventilations or other airway management, which will most likely be required, you must ensure that the airway is clear of any and all obstructions.

Subtest 6: Operations (30 items)

1. D. When approaching an intersection with a red light, you must always come to a complete stop, ensure that there is no oncoming traffic that has the right of way, and then proceed with caution through the red light. The majority of emergency vehicle crashes occur at intersections because the driver did not properly enter the intersection as described.

2. C. Considering that you can manage only one critical patient effectively per ambulance (with two medics), the most appropriate action is to call for an additional ambulance to respond to the scene. This must be accomplished as soon as you have determined that there are more patients than you can effectively manage.

3. B. Indications of a potentially unsafe scene include, but are certainly not limited to, the sound of breaking glass, a screaming individual, or gunfire. In cases such as these, the paramedic must not enter the scene until it has been secured by law enforcement. A patient's size does not indicate a potential for violence.

4. A. Once it has been identified that a patient is an organ donor, provided that obvious signs of death are not present (ie, decapitation, rigor mortis, dismemberment, etc), you should provide aggressive management and rapidly transport the patient to the hospital, where their organs potentially can be harvested.

5. B. Once you leave a carbon copy of a prehospital care report (PCR) form at the receiving facility, you cannot write anything else on the front of the form. Legally, this would make the original and the copy two separate documents, which could be easily scrutinized in a court of law. If further documentation is required after leaving the hospital, you should write on the reverse side of the form, or write a separate addendum, which becomes an official part of the PCR.

6. D. A mentally competent adult has the legal right to refuse care and to withdraw consent once it has been given. To further treat a mentally competent patient who withdraws consent could constitute assault, battery, or false imprisonment.

7. B. Negligence is defined as the failure to perform the accepted standard of care. Clearly, a patient involved in a significant motor vehicle crash would require full spinal immobilization, regardless of whether or not he or she is ambulatory on EMS arrival. Remember the "4 Ds" that are required to prove negligence: duty to act, duty not performed, direct harm, and disability to the patient.

8. B. When a patient demands that you provide care that is contraindicated for his or her condition, the best action to take is to contact medical control, apprise him or her of the situation, and seek further guidance.

9. D. One of the most effective ways for an EMS provider to allay his or her anxiety after a bad call is to talk with a fellow coworker, especially one who was involved in the call. This will allow for an immediate defusing and significantly minimizes the risk of further stress and anxiety.

10. C. Reassurance and a safe comfortable transport to the hospital are both very effective ways to reduce stress and anxiety in a patient. You should never lie to a patient about their potential condition. Clearly, a patient with a suspected acute myocardial infarction should be transported to the hospital via EMS, not by private vehicle.

11. D. The scoop stretcher, also called an orthopedic stretcher or split litter, is very effective in transporting patients with suspected hip or pelvic fractures. Its contoured design provides excellent support. Additionally, it is easier to manipulate a scoop stretcher in a house.

12. C. When managing a patient at the scene of a crime, the paramedic must provide care, while at the same time making every effort to avoid disturbing the scene or manipulating evidence. In this case, it would be most appropriate to have a police officer retrieve the knife as you continue to treat the patient.

13. A. A "do not resuscitate" (DNR) order must be validated by a physician. In cases where a DNR is presented, especially if the document is questionable, it is best to err on the side of providing basic life support until a physician advises you to cease resuscitative efforts. Remember, when in doubt, resuscitate.

14. C. Part of caring for a patient is determining what lead to the injury or illness, which is a part of the SAMPLE history. This can be accomplished by ascertaining whether or not any bystanders witnessed the event.

15. A. When communicating with a patient who is confused, you must constantly keep him or her aware of the surroundings, what happened, and where you are going. No matter how many times a patient asks you, you must repeat the truth each time.

16. B. Informed consent is defined as ensuring that the patient is aware of the care that is to be provided as well as the potential complications associated with the treatment. This will give the patient enough information to make an informed decision about his or her health care. Making patients aware of the complications of suggested treatment is just as important as making them aware of the complications of refusing care.

17. C. Educating the public is a crucial aspect of a successful illness and injury prevention program. When you are explaining the importance of early notification of EMS through 9–1–1, advise the audience that this is critical because early defibrillation is the key factor in the survival of out-of-hospital cardiac arrest patients.

18. B. Because rescue breathing is a procedure that must take place after an injury or illness has occurred, it is not a component of injury or illness prevention. The key is to provide information that would prevent you or the bystander from having to perform such procedures to begin with.

19. A. Proper technique when lifting a patient involves keeping your palms up whenever possible, which will prevent unnecessary stress and potential injury to the wrists. When lifting, you should always use the powerful muscles of your legs.

20. B. The Centers for Disease Control and Prevention (CDC) states that effective hand washing, especially in-between patients, is the most effective means of preventing the spread of disease. Adherence to body substance isolation precautions will minimize your risk of disease exposure. To protect yourself from infection if you are exposed, it is important to keep your immunizations current.

21. C. Considering that you and your partner's safety are of primary concern, the best approach to take in the situation where a patient is slumped over the steering wheel of his or her car is to approach the vehicle from the rear. Shining a light into the side view mirror will prevent the person from seeing you until you can determine that the patient is safe to contact. Unfortunately, it is common for people to fake illness or injury with the intent of hurting the responding personnel.

22. C. Whether you are lifting or moving patient with or without a carrying device, you should avoid twisting at the same time you move around corners. Failing to do so could result in injury to your back.

23. B. Immediately after using a needle or other sharps device (ie, starting an IV, giving an injection), you should place it in a puncture-proof container (usually red). Waiting until the end of a call to search the ambulance for needles may result in an accidental needle stick. Prefilled syringes should be disposed of as an entire unit, without removing the needle.

24. A. Recognizing and rewarding personnel with good performance, strict adherence to all system protocols, and finding solutions for identified problems are all vital components to any quality assurance program, with the ultimate goal being the provision of consistently high-quality patient care.

25. C. Whenever operating an ambulance, whether in an emergent or nonemergent mode, you must always drive with due regard for those around you. This means that you must be prepared for erratic movements of other drivers and never assume that they will see and/or hear you. The use of escorts is discouraged because of the risk of a "wake effect" collision, which occurs when a police officer or other escort clears a red light for you and then proceeds. Drivers may not be expecting a second response vehicle, thus leading to a crash. Siren use does not guarantee a safe response, and increased speed clearly increases the risk of a crash.

26. B. Your best protection from legal liability is to consistently provide a high standard of care to all patients, which includes performing thorough assessments, providing the appropriate management, and thoroughly documenting the case.

27. D. Gross negligence occurs when patient care suffers as a result of an inappropriate action or inaction made on the part of the EMT or paramedic, without any attempt at taking corrective action. An example of this is failing to check the batteries on a defibrillator at the start of a shift. Other mistakes can be construed as negligence; however, if the individual accused takes or attempts to take corrective action, the likelihood of being found guilty is minimized.

28. D. Communication with area hospitals to determine their capabilities is the responsibility of the transport officer. By identifying each hospital's capabilities, the transport officer can direct exiting ambulances from the mass-casualty scene to the most appropriate facility.

29. D. Peripherally inserted central venous lines of many types are frequently found in home health care patients receiving long-term medication therapy, such as chemotherapy for cancer. Relative to central lines, which are more stable and need to be changed less frequently, peripherally inserted IV lines, such as what is more commonly encountered in an acute care setting, is an infrequent finding in the patient who is in need of long-term care.

30. C. If you are unable to reach medical control and a procedure needs to be performed, the most appropriate action would be to follow standard protocols, which may or may not include performing the procedure. Protocols vary from system to system.

Practice Final Examination (180 items)

1. C. As respirations decrease in rate and depth (tidal volume), carbon dioxide is retained. This leads to an initial state of respiratory acidosis. If left untreated, metabolic acidosis will result as the cells of the body begin producing lactic and pyruvic acid secondary to anaerobic metabolism.

2. C. The most effective means of controlling this particular patient's airway, even though generally considered as a last resort, is with a needle cricothyrotomy. Nasotracheal intubation is contraindicated because the patient is apneic. Mandibular fractures make both endotracheal intubation and ventilations with a BVM device difficult because both techniques rely on a stable mandible.

3. B. After determining that a patient is apneic, you should provide two rescue breaths, with each breath performed over 1 second—enough to produce visible chest rise. After delivering two breaths, assess for the patient's pulse. If the patient is pulseless, begin CPR and analyze his or her cardiac rhythm as soon as possible. Immediate intubation should not be performed without a period of preoxygenation using basic means, such as a BVM or pocket facemask.

4. B. Meperidine hydrochloride is a potent narcotic analgesic and will respond to the administration of naloxone. Naloxone is a narcotic antagonist that binds to opiate receptor sites in the body, thus blocking the narcotic effects (CNS depression) of meperidine hydrochloride such as decreased respirations, pulse rate, and blood pressure.

5. D. Of the cardiac rhythms listed, atrial fibrillation is the only one that is irregularly irregular. In fact, atrial fibrillation is never seen as a regular rhythm. At a rate of less than 100 beats/min, atrial fibrillation is said to be controlled. Uncontrolled atrial fibrillation occurs when the ventricular rate exceeds 100 beats/min.

6. C. The quickest and most effective method for controlling severe bleeding is with the use of direct pressure. It this is unsuccessful, apply pressure to a proximal pressure point. Because of the anatomic location of this patient's injury (the groin), application of a tourniquet would be impractical and most likely ineffective. Therefore, if direct pressure and pressure point control are unsuccessful, you should consider locating the bleeding artery and applying digital pressure. After the bleeding has been controlled, begin shock treatment (ie, oxygen, elevation of lower extremities, rapid transport, IV therapy).

7. D. A weak, thready pulse corresponds with a low cardiac output state and hypotension, both of which are late signs of shock. A patient that is comatose is also in the later stages of shock because of cerebral hypoxia and hypercarbia. In the early stages of shock, respirations will increase (tachypnea) and become shallow (reduced tidal volume) in an attempt to increase the oxygen content of the blood.

8. B. Do not let a patient's stable blood pressure fool you because it could drop at any time. The most appropriate IV therapy for this patient would include at least one large-bore IV for the purpose of maintaining perfusion should the patient start to deteriorate. If the patient becomes unstable, a second IV will be needed.

9. C. Early defibrillation is critical to survival from sudden cardiac arrest (SCA) for several reasons: 1) The most frequent initial rhythm in witnessed SCA is ventricular fibrillation (VF), 2) early defibrillation has clearly shown to be effective in terminating VF, 3) the probability of successful defibrillation decreases rapidly over time, and 4) VF tends to deteriorate to asystole within a matter of a few minutes.

10. A. An epidural hemorrhage, which is usually the result of damage to the middle meningeal artery, produces a loss of consciousness immediately after impact, after which the patient typically has a brief return of consciousness. As the arterial bleeding begins to increase the pressure within the cranium, the patient rapidly lapses into a coma.

11. C. Trismus is defined as clenching of the teeth due to spasm of the jaw muscles; it is a common finding in patients with severe head trauma. To most effectively control the airway, patients with trismus often require rapid sequence intubation (RSI). The condition in which the pupils are unequal is called anisocoria. In the context of head trauma, anisocoria is an ominous sign and indicates significantly increased intracranial pressure.

12. B. Any patient that is threatening suicide should be assumed to have the potential of hurting others as well. In any case involving a psychiatric patient, the safety of you and your partner comes first.

13. C. Sinus bradycardia is probably one of the most over treated cardiac rhythms. Before you reach for atropine or a pacemaker, determine if the bradycardia is impairing the patient's hemodynamic status (ie, hypotension, altered mental state, etc). If so, atropine and/or use of a pacemaker would be indicated.

14. B. Infants and children usually have healthy hearts. Many cardiac arrests in children can be prevented by paying meticulous attention to their respiratory status; respiratory failure is usually what leads to cardiac arrest.

15. C. The pediatric dose of epinephrine when administered endotracheally is 0.1 mg/kg of a 1:1,000 solution (0.1 mL/kg).

16. C. Myxedema, a complication of hypothyroidism, results from a decrease in the production of thyroid hormones (T3 and T4). Since the thyroid regulates the metabolic rate and metabolism produces body heat, patients with myxedema are at risk for hypothermia.

17. B. Typically, when a swimmer becomes panicked, he or she starts swallowing large amounts of water. Even a small volume of aspirated water (fresh or salt) can cause laryngospasm, which leads to hypoxia and unconsciousness. As the hypoxia worsens, cardiac dysrhythmias can develop, which leads to cardiac arrest.

18. A. The patient's airway is rapidly swelling as evidenced by the markedly diminished breath sounds and loud inspiratory stridor. If the patient is not promptly intubated before the airway completely closes, you will have to perform a needle cricothyrotomy or the patient will die.

19. C. Because small children rely mainly on their pulse rate to maintain perfusion, bradycardia, if present, is an ominous sign indicating late hypoxia and requires immediate positive pressure ventilations. If the pulse rate falls below 60 beats/min, chest compressions must be initiated.

20. D. According to the 2005 Emergency Cardiac Care (ECC) guidelines, vasopressin, in a one-time dose of 40 units, can be given to replace the first or second dose of epinephrine for adult patients in cardiac arrest. There are no definitive data to support superiority of vasopressin over epinephrine; furthermore, the efficacy of vasopressin has not been established for pediatric cardiac arrest patients.

21. A. Following return of spontaneous circulation (ROSC), immediately reassess airway and breathing. If the patient remains apneic, ventilate at a rate of 10 to 12 breaths/min; hyperventilation should be avoided as this may impair venous return and cardiac output. Assess and support the patient's blood pressure; this may involve administering a fluid bolus or an inotropic agent (ie, dopamine). Since amiodarone was administered to the patient during the arrest, a maintenance infusion at 1 mg/min should be initiated in order to maintain a therapeutic blood level.

22. B. Because of the predominance of ventricular fibrillation in the majority of adult cardiac arrest patients, it must be emphasized to laypeople that early, effective CPR and defibrillation are the most critical interventions and have clearly demonstrated increased survival rates from cardiac arrest. Fibrinolytic drugs are contraindicated in patients with cardiac arrest. Early advanced care (ie, intubation, cardiac medications, etc) and rapid transport are clearly important to the patient's survival; however, the vast majority of patients who survive out-of-hospital cardiac arrest received early, effective CPR and prompt defibrillation.

23. D. As a paramedic, you have been educated on the appropriate doses of a wide array of medications, including morphine. If you receive an order that is contrary to what you were taught, especially when the order calls for five times the normal dose, you should advise the physician of this and ask him or her to clarify or repeat the order. If a physician orders you to administer a drug in an inappropriate dose and you carry out the order, you could be held equally liable for the consequences.

24. C. The quick look is only performed on patients in cardiac arrest to rapidly assess their need for defibrillation. Conscious patients should have the electrodes and leads placed to assess the rhythm.

25. A. Injuries that are close to the knee, as in the case of a distal femur fracture, should not have a traction splint applied, especially if the fracture is open with the femur protruding through the skin. Instead, the fracture should be covered with a sterile dressing and immobilized in the position found. Any action that could cause the femur to retract back into the thigh significantly increases the risk of infection.

26. C. Patients with respiratory difficulty and reduced tidal volume (shallow breathing) are not taking in sufficient amounts of air to support adequate oxygenation; therefore, ventilation assistance is required in order to restore tidal volume and minute volume. If the patient resists ventilation assistance, apply a nonrebreathing mask but be prepared to resume ventilation assistance if the patient's level of conscious deteriorates secondary to hypoxia and hypercarbia.

27. A. A patent airway is one that is free of obstructions and secretions. Gurgling respirations indicate fluid in the airway. Snoring respirations indicate partial obstruction by the tongue—the most common cause of airway obstruction in unresponsive patients. Inspiratory stridor indicates upper airway swelling. Cyanosis, although clearly a sign of hypoxia, is a relatively later finding. A patient who is coughing *forcefully* has a patent airway.

28. B. On arriving at the scene of any emergency (medical or trauma), you should always conduct a scene size-up. This begins by surveying the area to ensure that there are no dangers or hazards that would pose a threat to you or your crew. The presence of law enforcement at the scene does not automatically equate to a safe environment. Remember, the life you save may take your own.

29. C. After noting that the patient's level of consciousness is diminished, you must next ensure a patent airway. Since this is a trauma patient, the jaw-thrust maneuver must be used.

30. B. Respirations of 20 breaths/min and eupneic (normal) indicate that this patient is breathing adequately. On the basis of these findings, 100% supplemental oxygen should be applied using a nonrebreathing mask. The patient's breathing should be continuously monitored for signs of inadequacy, in which case assisted ventilations must be initiated.

31. B. The *rhythm* depicted is sinus tachycardia at a rate of approximately 100 to 110 beats/min. First-degree AV block is characterized by a PR interval that is greater than 0.20 seconds, the normal being 0.12 to 0.20 seconds (120 to 200 milliseconds). The fact that the patient does not have a pulse indicates pulseless electrical activity (PEA). *PEA is not a specific rhythm; it is a condition* in which a pulseless, apneic patient presents with an organized cardiac rhythm (except V-fib and pulseless V-tach).

32. B. After determining that the patient is in pulseless electrical activity (PEA), you should begin CPR as your partner prepares to secure the airway with an endotracheal tube.

33. C. Acidosis is a common cause of pulseless electrical activity (PEA). It should be assumed to exist to some degree in any cardiac arrest patient. Remember, the initial treatment for acidosis—regardless of the underlying cause—is increased ventilation, not sodium bicarbonate! Other common causes of PEA include hypovolemia, hypoxia, hypo- or hyperkalemia, hypothermia, toxins (ie, drug overdose), cardiac tamponade, tension pneumothorax, trauma, and pulmonary or coronary thrombosis.

34. C. Diabetic ketoacidosis, also referred to as diabetic coma, is characterized by hyperglycemia, polyuria (excessive urination), polydipsia (excessive thirst), and polyphagia (excessive hunger). Other findings include warm, dry skin, dehydration, and deep, rapid respirations (Kussmaul respirations).

35. B. As with any patient, preventing further harm or injury is your initial priority of patient care. In a patient with a swollen, painful deformity, the injury should be manually stabilized until completely immobilized, with the assessment of distal pulses before and after immobilization.

36. B. Because of the excess fluid within the pericardial sac, cardiac contraction is restricted, which causes a drop in the systolic pressure, and full relaxation is inhibited causing an increase in the diastolic pressure. The difference between the systolic and diastolic pressures is called the pulse pressure, which becomes narrowed with a pericardial tamponade. A blood pressure of 90/70 mm Hg has a pulse pressure of only 20 mm Hg, which is less than any of the other values listed.

37. A. As soon as the baby's head has delivered, you must immediately suction the oropharynx (mouth) first, and then the nose. It is extremely important to clear the baby's airway of fetal lung fluid prior to it taking its first breath. Once the baby has completely delivered, suctioning of the mouth and nose is repeated. Drying, warming, and stimulating the baby to breathe if needed are also carried out.

38. D. Fortunately, most children with febrile seizures do well and very few require hospitalization. General care for the child after the seizure has occurred is mainly supportive, consisting of monitoring the airway and offering the child oxygen. Diazepam is not indicated unless the child is experiencing a prolonged seizure. Cooling of a child with a fever who has just had a seizure should be avoided because it may cause the child to shiver, resulting in an abrupt rise in body temperature and the possibility of another seizure.

39. B. A delay in capillary refill is a very reliable indicator of early shock in children younger than age 6 years. Remember that factors such as cold temperatures can influence capillary refill time. A weak, rapid pulse is a late sign of shock in any patient. A slow, bounding pulse would be more indicative of closed head injury with increased intracranial pressure. Confusion and anxiety are not reliable parameters in a 2-year-old child because they are difficult to assess.

40. A. Body substance isolation precautions require gloves only when caring for a patient with AIDS who is not actively coughing. If there is any chance of body fluid splatter (ie, coughing up blood), a mask and gown would be needed. One factor to consider is to place a mask on the patient, which will serve to protect him or her from any illnesses that you might have.

41. D. When in doubt, resuscitate. You should not withhold resuscitative efforts while awaiting proper documentation. Even after such paperwork is provided, you must notify medical control and seek advice as to whether or not you should proceed with the resuscitation or terminate your efforts.

42. D. Angioneurotic edema, caused by the release of histamines, is the result of vascular fluid leakage into the subcutaneous layers of the skin. It is prominent in the face and neck area in patients with severe allergic reactions and can pose a significant threat to the airway.

43. B. The patient's symptoms are consistent with a space-occupying intracranial lesion such as a neoplasm (tumor or growth), which typically presents with a headache, visual disturbances, and other symptoms that progressively worsen over a period of several months. Subdural hemorrhages commonly present with symptoms within 12 to 24 hours following head trauma. An epidural hematoma presents with symptoms immediately following head injury and causes rapid deterioration. Patients with bacterial meningitis also experience a rapid progression of symptoms.

44. C. Central cyanosis and a pulse rate of less than 100 beats/min are both indicators of hypoxia in the newborn, which must be treated with immediate positive pressure ventilations. Chest compressions must be started if the pulse rate falls below 60 beats/min.

45. C. Although the patient is conscious and able to converse, she is clearly showing signs of hypoxia (anxiety, an oxygen saturation level of 90%, rapid pulse). Therefore, she should be given 100% supplemental oxygen as soon as possible. You must be prepared to assist with ventilations should her level of consciousness deteriorate or her breathing becomes inadequate.

46. A. Since this rhythm has narrow QRS complexes and a rate greater than 150 beats/min, it should be interpreted as supraventricular tachycardia (SVT), which means that its site of origin is above (supra) the level of the ventricles. SVT can be either atrial or junctional in origin. Atrial fibrillation is characterized by an irregularly irregular rhythm and no discernable P waves. Atrial flutter is characterized by flutter (F) waves that resemble a saw tooth. Ventricular tachycardia (V-tach), in contrast to SVT, is characterized by wide (greater than 0.12 seconds) QRS complexes.

47. D. Because of the patient's low blood pressure and obvious respiratory distress, her condition is considered unstable. Therefore, you should consider sedation (monitor the blood pressure carefully) and cardiovert the rhythm beginning with 100 joules.

48. D. Recalling the patient's initial statement and presentation, she told you that she was suddenly awaked with a smothering feeling. This is referred to as paroxysmal nocturnal dyspnea (PND). A combination of PND as well as the dried blood on her lips (probably secondary to coughing up blood-tinged sputum) is consistent with left-sided heart failure, in which stroke volume (the amount of blood ejected from the left ventricle) is decreased secondary to myocardial weakening or damage. This results in backing up of blood into the lungs, causing pulmonary edema.

49. C. The patient has most likely had an acute myocardial infarction. However, he also is showing signs of hypoperfusion, which indicates that a significant degree of myocardium has been destroyed. Hypoperfusion of cardiac origin is referred to as cardiogenic shock and has a mortality rate of approximately 80%.

50. A. Because of its positive inotropic effect of increasing myocardial contractility, dopamine is the drug of choice for non-hypovolemic shock (eg, cardiogenic shock) and may improve perfusion. Typically, dopamine for cardiogenic shock is started at 2 µg/kg/min and titrated upwards as needed to improve blood pressure and perfusion. High-dose dopamine (> 10 µg/kg/min) has more of a vasopressor effect, which results in systemic vasoconstriction. Clearly, nitroglycerin is contraindicated in any patient with shock; its potent vasodilatory effects would further lower the patient's blood pressure and worsen his condition.

51. C. Use of a pharyngeal tracheal lumen airway, as well as a Combitube, is contraindicated in children younger than age 14 years. It is also contraindicated in caustic ingestions and in patients who are less than 5′ tall, have known esophageal diseases, or have a gag reflex.

52. A. Because the endotracheal tube is advanced when the patient inhales (the vocal cords are open at their widest), blind nasotracheal intubation is contraindicated in apneic patients.

53. D. Clearly, prevention is the best medicine. Recognizing early signs of shock, minimizing on scene time, and recognizing patients with a significant MOI are all critical to the outcome of the patient, but these could be non-issues if the injury were prevented in the first place.

54. B. Typically, when an adult is struck by an automobile, his or her initial instinct is to turn away from the car. The initial point of impact is generally to the lateral aspect of the body. The patient is then thrown onto the hood and/or windshield, and then propelled away from the automobile.

55. B. The blast from an explosion causes a wave of pressure. This wave causes the initial trauma to the patient, usually in the form of burns and barotrauma. Secondary injuries occur when the patient is struck by flying debris, and tertiary injuries result from the patient being thrown into fixed structures or other hard surfaces.

56. A. There are approximately 1 million patients with various malignancies (cancers) receiving home health care in this country today. Most cancer patients prefer to die in the privacy of their own homes. Additionally, lengthy hospital stays for treatment that could be just as easily rendered at home are astronomical in cost.

57. D. Bronchopulmonary dysplasia (BPD) is a lung disease that typically affects low birth weight infants and is characterized by chronic respiratory distress and frequent lower respiratory tract infections. The basic underlying etiology behind BPD is a deficiency of pulmonary surfactant at birth. Surfactant acts to lubricate the alveolar walls, allowing them to expand and recoil normally.

58. B. Remember that you must always document factual findings, not your own opinion. Documenting statements that are reflective of your personal opinion could lead to allegations of libel against you.

59. C. General care for a pit viper bite includes placing the patient in a supine position, keeping the affected extremity lower than the level of the heart, and immobilizing the extremity. Additionally, an IV should be initiated and the patient promptly transported to the hospital for treatment with antivenin. Ice is never applied to a snake bite because it is thought to increase the toxicity of the venom.

60. D. People who have recently experienced a major negative life change, such as financial hardship, loss of a loved one or a job, and those who are having marital problems are at a very high risk for suicide.

61. A. Remember that your personal safety comes first in all cases. You should be concerned with avoiding confrontation, providing safe transport, and managing any concomitant medical problems when managing a patient with a behavioral crisis, but do not let these supercede your own safety.

62. B. At the scene of a crime, you should provide needed care, while at the same time manipulating the scene as little as possible. In the case of a decapitation, the patient is obviously deceased; therefore, there should be no need to make any contact with the patient.

63. A. The EMS medical director plays an active role in establishing the paramedic's scope of practice, participating in the quality assurance process, and ensuring that all personnel are adequately trained and educated. The medical director, unless he or she wishes to directly observe the paramedic in the field, usually does not respond to the scene.

64. C. Even though the paramedic performed the skill appropriately and in the correct circumstance, advanced life support providers are not allowed to function as such when not on duty and/or affiliated with an EMS system under the auspices of a medical director. Doing so is considered practicing medicine without a license.

65. B. On the basis of the patient history and physical findings, this case is consistent with an anxiety attack and hyperventilation syndrome. These patients initially need emotional support and respiratory coaching. If the patient's respirations do not slow down after a reasonable period of coaching, you must assume the presence of another underlying cause, such as hypoxia and administer 100% oxygen. Rebreathing into a paper bag or any other action that causes the patient to rebreathe his or her own carbon dioxide (face mask with minimal oxygen flow) is no longer the standard of care. There are many other causes of hyperventilation other than stress and anxiety.

66. A. Gasping for air and a pulse oximeter reading of 84% are clear signs that this patient is not breathing adequately; therefore, he will require some form of ventilatory assistance, such as a BVM device with 100% supplemental oxygen. The fact that he is awake negates the use of an oral airway. Should the patient deteriorate further, he may require endotracheal intubation.

67. C. Beta-agonists, such as albuterol or metaproterenol sulfate, are generally given via a nebulizer for patients with reactive airway diseases (ie, asthma, bronchitis, etc) to promote bronchodilation and improve breathing effort. A patient with bronchoconstriction, as evidenced by wheezing, must never be given a beta-blocker as this would result in worsened lower airway constriction and could lead to respiratory failure.

68. D. Patients with asthma have two problems: bronchoconstriction and hypoxia; therefore, the goals of management are to relieve the bronchospasm and improve ventilation and oxygenation. Dehydration tends to occur in patients with asthma because of mucous plug formation and drying of the lower airway (children especially); therefore, fluid hydration may be required.

69. C. Acetylcholinesterase is like the body's "internal atropine" in that it regulates the production of acetylcholine. Inhibition of this chemical would result in signs of severe increased parasympathetic tone (excessive salivation, lacrimation, and urination). Organophosphates tend to significantly inhibit the production of acetylcholinesterase and may require large amounts of atropine to reverse this effect.

70. D. Amitriptyline hydrochloride, a tricyclic antidepressant (TCA), should be managed, among other modalities, with sodium bicarbonate which alkalinizes the urine and promotes the excretion of the drug via the kidneys. Diazepam is a benzodiazepine and would not respond to naloxone. Flumazenil, which reverses the effects of benzodiazepines, should never be given to patients who have overdosed with both TCAs and benzodiazepines as it may precipitate seizures. Additionally, this patient will require ventilatory assistance.

71. B. First secure a patent airway (jaw-thrust maneuver in trauma patients), clear the airway (suction as needed), and then provide management based on the adequacy of the patient's breathing.

72. C. The Parkland formula, which is used to determine how much IV crystalloid fluid a severely burned patient should receive within the first 24 hours following the burn, is calculated as follows:

4 mL × patient's weight in kilograms × percentage of body surface area (BSA) burned

On the basis of the above formula, a 160-lb (73 kg [160 4 2.2 5 73]) should receive 11,680 mL of IV crystalloid fluid within the first 24 hours following the burn:

4 mL × 73 (kg) × 40 (% BSA burned) = 11,680 mL

The Parkland formula further states that half of the 24-hour fluid amount should be given within the first 8 hours following the burn. Therefore, the calculation continues as follows:

11,680 mL (24-hour fluid amount) ÷ 2 = 5,840 mL (8-hour fluid amount)

Thus, if 5,840 mL is to be delivered over 8 hours, the patient should receive 730 mL of IV crystalloid per hour, as follows:

5,840 mL ÷ 8 = 730 mL

73. C. A common cause of death in patients with extensive burns, especially full-thickness burns, is swelling and closure of the airway. You must constantly monitor the patient for signs of swelling/closure, which include singed nasal hairs, a brassy cough, hoarseness, stridor, and progressive respiratory distress. In addition to monitoring the airway, the patient must be protected from hypothermia. A needle cricothyrotomy may be indicated should you be unable to intubate the patient.

74. A. One of the most effective ways to reduce stress and anxiety in a bystander at the scene of an emergency is to assign him or her minor, nonpatient care-related tasks. This may involve activities such as providing rescuers with water or other needed supplies. The goal is to occupy the bystander's mind and make him or her feel as though they are helping. It is not safe to tell an obviously upset bystander to go home because these people deserve appropriate care and attention as well. Functions such as crowd and traffic control are responsibilities of law enforcement.

75. B. Battery is defined as touching the patient without his or her expressed consent. You should never assume that a patient will readily accept your treatment; therefore, you must apprise them of what you intend to do prior to carrying out the task.

76. B. Any patient that refuses EMS care must be informed of the potential consequences of refusal. The most direct approach is to advise the patient that their condition could ultimately result in death. This ensures that the patient is aware of the potential worst-case scenario. If the patient still refuses, is of sound body and mind, and is willing to take that risk, there is little else you can do. Be sure to carefully document all attempts made by you to convince the patient to allow treatment and/or transport.

77. C. When assessing the chest of a trauma patient in the rapid trauma assessment, you should note any deformities, contusions, abrasions, penetrating injuries, burns, tenderness, lacerations, and swelling/symmetry of the chest wall (DCAP-BTLS). Further assessment should include auscultation of breath sounds and heart tones.

78. C. According to the American Heart Association, patients with *unwitnessed out-of-hospital cardiac arrest* have better survival rates after receiving about 2 minutes of CPR before defibrillation than those who received immediate defibrillation—especially when the EMS call-to-arrival interval is greater than 4 to 5 minutes. The patient in this scenario did not receive bystander CPR, and the EMS crew arrived approximately 8 minutes after his collapse. After 2 minutes (5 cycles) of CPR, the patient's cardiac rhythm should be analyzed. If V-fib or pulseless V-tach is present, defibrillate one time with 360 joules followed immediately by CPR.

79. D. Current Emergency Cardiac Care (ECC) guidelines state that the initial dose of amiodarone for ventricular fibrillation (V-fib) or pulseless ventricular tachycardia (V-tach) is 300 mg via rapid IV push. *Administer the drug without interrupting CPR* and then reassess the patient's cardiac rhythm after 2 minutes of CPR. If V-fib or pulseless V-tach persists, defibrillate one time with 360 joules followed by immediate resumption of CPR.

80. C. Because bleeding into the retroperitoneal space may not produce the obvious signs of abdominal injury (ie, distention, rigidity, bruising, etc), trauma patients with unexplained shock (hypoperfusion) should be assumed to have an intra-abdominal hemorrhage. The retroperitoneal space is a common area for hidden bleeding.

81. A. Although there is still controversy regarding the use of the PASG, the general medical community agrees that the PASG is clearly indicated for patients with pelvic fractures and/or bilateral femur fractures with hypotension. The PASG is not indicated for patients with any injury that is above the level of the last rib or with open abdominal injuries. The PASG should never be placed on a patient with congestive heart failure and pulmonary edema or on patients with cardiogenic shock.

82. D. Patient assessment involves simple patient questioning techniques. You should always ask open-ended questions. Asking a leading question, such as "Do you have sharp chest pain?" will often times lead the patient to say "yes," even though that is not the true quality of his or her pain. Allow the patient to use his or her own words when describing symptoms.

83. C. The American Heart Association mnemonic "MONA" represents the initial management for patients with suspected cardiac chest pain. Although it does not represent the correct order in which the treatment should be rendered, it is a good mnemonic to remember. The appropriate order of medications is oxygen, aspirin (160 to 325 mg), nitrogylcerin (0.4 mg up to 3 times), and morphine (2 to 4 mg) if the nitroglycerin does not relieve the chest pain. Pain relief is extremely important in a patient with an acute myocardial infarction because it reduces anxiety and subsequent oxygen consumption and demand.

84. C. Energy settings for manual biphasic defibrillators are device-specific—typically 120 joules (rectilinear) or 150 joules (truncated). However, if the appropriate initial energy setting is unknown, the 2005 Emergency Cardiac Care (ECC) guidelines recommend defibrillation with 200 joules. For subsequent shocks, use the same or higher energy setting. Whether you are using a monophasic or biphasic manual defibrillator, you should only perform 1 shock, followed immediately by CPR. The initial 3-shock sequence is no longer recommended.

85. A. Thorough objective documentation of the scene and examination findings is vital in cases of suspected abuse. By law, you must report any and all cases of suspected abuse to the proper authority, which is the physician at the receiving hospital, who in turn has a legal obligation to notify child protective services (CPS). You should never confront or accuse the parents or caregivers of abuse because this could result in slander on your part if you are wrong. In addition, you must obtain consent from at least one parent prior to transporting the child, otherwise you may be held accountable for kidnapping.

86. A. If you must restrain a violent patient, you must ensure the presence of at least four people (one for each extremity). The patient should be restrained in the prone position with someone constantly talking to the patient through the process. The use of "reasonable" force definitely applies when restraining a patient. If you use unnecessary force when restraining the patient and he or she is in the prone position, compromise of the airway could occur. This is called positional asphyxia. You must ensure that the patient is restrained in a manner where the airway is not compromised and you can easily assess it.

87. B. Children older than 1 month should receive fluid resuscitation at a rate of 20 mL/kg, followed by a reassessment. According to the current AHA and American Academy of Pediatrics (AAP) guidelines, neonates (younger than 1 month) should receive fluids at a rate of 10 mL/kg. Remember that the most common error made with fluid resuscitation in children is not giving enough fluids.

88. C. Whether CPR is in progress on your arrival or not, you must still perform the initial survey of the ABCs, which includes determining the presence of cardiac arrest. Many times, CPR will be performed on those who do not require it. Once cardiac arrest is confirmed, your next priority is to perform a quick look with the defibrillator paddles to assess the need for defibrillation.

89. D. The rhythm shown is a sinus rhythm with first-degree AV block. Even after pulselessness has been confirmed and CPR initiated, the pulse must be assessed if this or any other potentially perfusing rhythm appears on the cardiac monitor.

90. C. Once vascular access has been obtained, the first drug and dose given to all patients in cardiac arrest—regardless of the rhythm on the cardiac monitor—is epinephrine 1 mg (1:10,000) repeated every 3 to 5 minutes. You may consider a *one-time* dose of vasopressin (40 units) to replace the first or second dose of epinephrine. Higher doses of epinephrine may be necessary if special circumstances exist (ie, severe beta-blocker toxicity). Consult with medical control as needed.

91. D. Immediately after placement of the endotracheal tube, you must inflate the distal cuff with 5 to 10 mL of air, remove the syringe, and then attach the BVM device for ventilations and confirmation of correct tube placement. The rationale for immediate cuff inflation is to prevent regurgitation and subsequent aspiration that can be associated with the intubation procedure.

92. A. In patients with cardiogenic pulmonary edema (ie, congestive heart failure), morphine sulfate causes systemic pooling of blood which increases venous capacitance and decreases preload (the volume of blood returned to the right atrium). The net effect is to minimize the volume of fluid that accumulates in the lungs. Note that morphine is not a diuretic and will not remove fluid from the body. This is accomplished by administering furosemide, which is also given to patients in congestive heart failure.

93. D. As the right side of the heart fails, blood is not effectively ejected into the pulmonary circuit; therefore, it backs up beyond the right atrium and into the systemic venous system. This is most noticeable by the presence of engorged or distended jugular veins. Orthopnea, nocturnal dyspnea, and coughing up blood-tinged sputum are indicators of left-sided heart failure as they all indicate fluid in the lungs.

94. B. Patients with atrial fibrillation are commonly prescribed digoxin and warfarin sodium, which is a blood thinner. As the atria fibrillate, blood has the tendency to stagnate and form microemboli that can pass into a major artery (ie, pulmonary, cerebral, coronary, etc) and cause a blockage.

95. C. Since oxygen has already been administered to this patient and your partner is attaching the ECG leads, your next most appropriate action is to administer 160 to 325 mg of aspirin. The next drug of choice would be nitroglycerin, followed by morphine IV if the nitroglycerin fails to relieve the pain.

96. A. Enalapril maleate (Vasotec) is an ACE (angiotensin-converting enzyme) inhibitor that is used to treat hypertension. Angiotensin, which is produced in the kidneys, is a potent vasoconstrictor. By inhibiting its release, the blood pressure can be kept under control. Propranolol hydrochloride (Inderal) and metoprolol tartrate (Lopressor) are beta-blockers. Nifedipine (Procardia) and diltiazem (Cardizem) are calcium channel blockers. An example of a parasympathetic blocker is atropine sulfate.

97. C. This patient is in ventricular tachycardia (V-tach). Furthermore, he is hemodynamically unstable (eg, confusion, hypotension). Therefore, the most appropriate treatment is to consider sedation (ie, Versed, Valium) and then perform synchronized cardioversion at 100 joules. Amiodarone would be an appropriate intervention if the patient was stable. Vagal maneuvers and adenosine are appropriate for stable patients with narrow complex tachycardias (eg, SVT). Fluid boluses will likely not improve the patient's blood pressure; his hypotension is the result of inadequate ventricular filling and decreased cardiac output due to his cardiac rhythm—not hypovolemia.

98. A. Any time a patient's condition suddenly deteriorates, you must immediately repeat the initial assessment, which begins by ensuring a patent airway and then providing management that is appropriate for the patient's condition.

99. B. Agonal respirations (occasional gasping breaths) are ineffective and are managed as if the patient were apneic. Your most appropriate action is to provide immediate rescue breathing through either a BVM device or a pocket mask device. Clearly, this patient will require intubation but not before a 2- to 3-minute period of preoxygenation.

100. B. You have witnessed this patient's deterioration to coarse ventricular fibrillation; therefore, you should defibrillate one time with 360 joules followed by immediate CPR. Perform 5 cycles of CPR (about 2 minutes) and then reassess the patient's cardiac rhythm. If the patient is still in ventricular fibrillation, defibrillate again with 360 joules and immediately resume CPR.

101. C. Oxygen that is delivered nasally, especially over a prolonged period of time, can cause drying and irritation of the nasal mucosa; therefore, an oxygen humidifier should be attached.

102. D. A pH of 7.1 represents an acidodic state. An elevated PCO_2 indicates carbon dioxide retention; therefore, without knowing the $NaHCO_3^-$ (Bicarb) level, you have no choice but to call this a respiratory acidosis. Alkalosis of any kind is quickly ruled out because of the low pH.

103. B. Acidosis, regardless of the underlying cause, is managed initially by increasing the depth (tidal volume) and rate of ventilations, especially with this patient, who is clearly retaining too much carbon dioxide. If the bicarb level was known and the base deficit could be calculated, sodium bicarbonate therapy would be appropriate because it should be given in patients with documented metabolic acidosis; but remember, ventilations first.

104. A. The patient's blood pressure and pulse (which should be fast) are not consistent with hypovolemic shock. Taking into consideration the mechanism of injury, the fact that she is motionless (from spinal injury), and the lack of tachycardia, neurogenic shock should be suspected. This occurs when injury to the spinal cord damages or destroys the spinal nerves that send messages to the sympathetic nervous system, thereby inhibiting the release of catecholamines (epinephrine and norepinephrine), which result in tachycardia and diaphoresis.

105. C. Sympathetic nervous system stimulation causes increased secretion of sweat, which explains why patients in shock are diaphoretic. Peripheral vasoconstriction results in shunting of blood to the central organs and gives the skin a pale appearance because of the absence of peripheral blood flow.

106. B. Men or women who are abused typically do not report the crime to the authorities because of the fear of repercussion from the abuser. It is not that the individuals do not want to come forward; they are simply scared.

107. B. The patient is in hypovolemic shock because of a pelvic fracture with internal bleeding. Beta-blocking medications (propranolol hydrochloride, metoprolol tartrate, etc) inhibit the sympathetic discharge of catecholamines that is commonly seen in patients with shock; therefore, epinephrine and norepinephrine are not released and diaphoresis and tachycardia do not occur.

108. C. Endotracheal intubation typically causes stimulation of the sympathetic nervous system; therefore, it is common to see increases in both the pulse rate and blood pressure during the procedure. This is usually handled well in most patients, provided that they do not have concomitant head injury with increased intracranial pressure. In cases such as this, lidocaine can be given, which transiently blunts the sudden rise in intracranial pressure during intubation.

109. B. Cardiomyopathy is a progressive weakening of the myocardium. This condition is commonly the result of chronic hypertension or a history of multiple myocardial infarctions. An enlarged myocardium is called cardiomegaly.

110. D. Side effects of the administration of atropine sulfate include thirst, dry mouth, pupillary dilation, tachycardia, hypertension, and urinary retention, especially in older men who have enlarged prostate glands.

111. A. Selective beta$_2$-adrenergic agonists, such as albuterol and metaproterenol sulfate, affect the lungs and result in bronchodilation; therefore, their use is indicated for patients with reactive airway diseases and accompanying bronchospasm. Selective beta$_1$-agonists possess an effect on the heart, resulting in increased contractility (inotropy) and increased pulse rate.

112. C. With an initial dose of 6 mg, followed by a dose of 12 mg that may be repeated once, the dose of adenosine should not exceed a cumulative dose of 30 mg when treating a narrow complex tachycardia in an adult.

113. B. Sympathomimetic medications such as epinephrine and norepinephrine cause increases in both myocardial oxygen demand and consumption. If given to patients who are suffering from hypoxia or acute myocardial infarction, this effect can result in cardiac arrhythmias. Therefore, any patient who is administered a sympathomimetic drug should be on a cardiac monitor.

114. C. The progressive lengthening of the PR interval until a P wave is blocked (not followed by a QRS complex) makes this cardiac rhythm a type I second-degree AV block, also referred to as "Wenckebach." This block represents a progressive delay at the AV node until an electrical impulse is completely blocked from entering the ventricles.

115. A. Croup, or laryngotracheobronchitis, is a viral upper respiratory illness that typically affects children between the ages of 6 months and 4 years. It is characterized by a low-grade fever (common with a viral infection) and respiratory distress, and typically has a slow onset of symptoms. Epiglottitis, which is a bacterial infection, produces a rapid onset of high fever, difficulty breathing, and is accompanied by signs such as drooling, difficulty swallowing, and inspiratory stridor. Epiglottitis is not as common in children as it used to be, but when it occurs, it commonly affects children between the ages of 3 to 7 years.

116. A. A pattern of irregular breathing that varies in depth and rate with sudden periods of apnea is referred to as Biot's respirations. This respiratory pattern is commonly seen in patients with increased intracranial pressure either from closed head trauma or hemorrhagic stroke. Clearly, patients displaying this respiratory pattern need ventilatory assistance.

117. B. Pulsus paradoxus, which is defined as a 10- to 15-mm Hg drop in blood pressure during inspiration, is seen in patients with pericardial tamponade (as a later sign), asthma, and COPD. In pericardial tamponade, the heart is already restricted from contracting and when the lungs enlarge during inhalation; this puts even more pressure on the heart and literally stops it until the patient exhales. You can assess for pulsus paradoxus by palpating the radial pulse and noting that it disappears when the patient inhales and returns when the patient exhales. This is the equivalent to a 10- to 15-mm Hg drop in blood pressure.

118. D. In patients with severe hypothermia (core body temperature less than 86°F [30°C]) with accompanying cardiac arrest, management includes CPR, intubation, and limiting defibrillation to one attempt if the patient is in ventricular fibrillation or pulseless ventricular tachycardia. Cardiac medications should be withheld at this point for two reasons: 1) the patient's metabolic rate is too slow to distribute the drugs, and 2) medications can accumulate to toxic levels in the severely hypothermic patient, which can result in negative consequences as the patient is rewarmed.

119. C. Signs and symptoms of HIV/AIDS include weight loss, which gives the patient an emaciated appearance, persistent fever, night sweats, fatigue, and purplish blotches on the skin, which are malignant lesions called Kaposi's sarcoma.

120. A. Rales, which are fine, moist, thin sounds that are difficult to auscultate, represent fluid in the small lower airways and are indicative of early pulmonary edema (ie, congestive heart failure). Rhonchi are loud rattling sounds that can often be heard without a stethoscope and are indicative of fluid in the larger airways (ie, severe pulmonary edema).

121. C. Patients younger than age 18 years cannot legally give consent for treatment, nor can they legally refuse transport. Exceptions to this include female minors who are emancipated or married. Prior to treating and/or transporting a child, you must obtain consent from at least one parent. A unique challenge is presented by patients who awaken after the administration of glucose. Provided that they are of sound mind and body at the time of refusal, they can legally refuse further treatment and/or transport.

122. B. The "Golden Hour" is crucial to the survival of critically injured patients. The "Platinum Ten" minutes represents the maximum amount of time that should be spent at the scene with these patients. We must remember that we are not definitive care providers. Our job is to recognize injuries, stabilize the patient, and provide transport to a facility where the injuries can be repaired surgically.

123. C. A sudden onset of difficulty breathing with pleuritic chest pain, especially in a patient with a recent history of hospitalization or prolonged bed rest in which blood tends to stagnate in the lower extremities and thus forms thrombi that can break free and lodge in a pulmonary artery, are all consistent with an acute pulmonary embolism. The patient's cyanosis, diaphoresis, and low oxygen saturation level indicate a significant degree of hypoxemia.

124. B. When assessing a patient's pulse during your baseline vital signs, you are noting the rate, regularity, and quality (strong, bounding, thready, etc). These parameters can give you a good idea as to the patient's overall perfusion status, especially when assessing a critically ill or injured patient.

125. C. There is little that the paramedic can do to have a definitive effect on a patient's underlying psychiatric illness; therefore, the ultimate goal is to provide transportation to the hospital while ensuring the safety of both yourself and the patient. In cases such as these, the assistance of law enforcement may be needed.

126. A. The "hunger" center of the hypothalamus promotes eating. Among many other functions, the hypothalamus regulates body temperature, assists in the regulatory control of the pituitary gland, and promotes urine release from the bladder. Influencing the patient's respirations is a function of the pons, which is a portion of the brainstem. Maintenance of equilibrium and balance are functions of the cerebellum, and the control of emotions and level of awareness are functions of the cerebrum, which is the largest portion of the brain, commonly referred to as the gray mater.

127. C. The patient is obviously experiencing a significant degree of respiratory distress and is hypoxic, as evidenced by his extreme restlessness. In cases such as this, your most appropriate action is to attempt to calm the patient and offer oxygen with a less oppressive device, such as a nasal cannula. Should the patient's level of consciousness decrease, you will most likely have to initiate positive pressure ventilations. CNS depressants, such as diazepam, should never be given to hypoxic patients with respiratory distress as it may cause respiratory arrest.

128. B. Gravida refers to the number of times the patient has been pregnant, and para refers to the number of live births. Gravida-4 indicates that this patient has been pregnant four times and para-3 indicates that she has three living children. If this baby delivers alive, she will become para-4.

129. B. With the exception of crowning, one of the most reliable indicators of imminent delivery is when the mother feels the urge to push. This indicates that the baby is in the birth canal and is resting on top of the rectum. Rupture of the amniotic sac indicates that delivery is near but not necessarily imminent. There is no correlation between the length of labor with her last child and imminent delivery with this child. Mothers who have had multiple children can remain in the second stage of labor for many hours, and those who are pregnant for the first time can progress through all stages of labor in less than 2 hours.

130. D. Positioning the mother in the left lateral recumbent position will take the pressure of the gravid uterus off of the inferior vena cava and improve cardiac output. Placing the patient in a supine position can result in supine hypotensive syndrome and subsequent shock, which would be detrimental to both mother and baby.

131. A. During transport, you should administer oxygen via either a nasal cannula or nonrebreathing mask, which will serve to keep both mother and baby well oxygenated. Follow local protocols for the most appropriate oxygen therapy. Two large-bore IVs are not indicated unless the mother is showing signs of shock or has severe vaginal bleeding; however, if time permits you should initiate one IV of normal saline solution at a keep-open rate. Clearly, internal vaginal examinations are beyond the scope of practice of the paramedic and will not provide any information that you do not already know. You should elevate the lower extremities if the mother is showing signs of shock.

132. D. If en route to the hospital the mother begins to deliver the baby, as evidenced by crowning, you should first tell the driver to stop the ambulance immediately and assist you in the back with the delivery. Never attempt to deliver a baby in the back of a moving ambulance as it is extremely unsafe.

133. B. A severe headache and vomiting that progressively worsens could indicate a subdural hemorrhage; therefore, the most important question to ask the patient is if he has experienced any recent head injury, even as far back as a week. Subdural hematomas are the result of venous bleeding and can be insidious in their presentation, with symptoms appearing several days after the initial injury. Hypertension is highly unlikely in a 16-year-old child, and meningitis is not a hereditary disease.

134. B. A toddler is defined as a child who is between the ages of 1 and 3 years. It is at this point where they are upwardly mobile and frequently get into things that they shouldn't, hence the advent of the child cabinet locks and outlet plug covers. An infant is from age 1 month to 1 year. A preschooler is from 3 to 5 years of age. A child is older than age 5 years.

135. C. Tachycardia is a common response of the child to many factors, both intrinsic and extrinsic. It is very common to see both tachycardia and tachypnea in response to fever. Flushing (redness) of the skin is also common. Small children cannot readily shiver as older children and adults can. This puts them in a high-risk category for hypothermia.

136. B. The oculomotor nerve, which is one of the 12 cranial nerves, arises from the midbrain and exits the brain to each eye. It controls the pupil's response to light. Damage to or pressure on this nerve will cause the pupils to dilate and take on the typical "blown" appearance. Common causes of this include increased intracranial pressure, stroke (both ischemic and hemorrhagic), and cerebral hypoxia.

137. C. When the initial assessment and management of an unresponsive medical patient is complete, the next step is to perform a rapid assessment. This step is identical to the rapid trauma assessment performed on a critically injured patient. The purpose of the rapid assessment is to further assess for and manage immediate life threats. Responsive medical patients usually have a focused physical exam that is based on their chief complaint.

138. D. Carbon monoxide (CO) binds to the hemoglobin molecule and inhibits the oxygen carrying ability of the blood. CO has an affinity for hemoglobin that is 200 times greater than that of oxygen. Cyanide blocks the uptake of oxygen at the cellular level. Both result in inadequate oxygenation and cellular death if left untreated.

139. B. First of all, you have to estimate the child's weight based on his age:
age in years × 2 + 8 = weight in kilograms
On the basis of the above formula, a typical 6-year-old child would weigh 20 kg. Fluid boluses for children are at 20 mL/kg; therefore, this child must receive 400 mL of crystalloid per bolus.

140. D. The reticular activating system (RAS), which is located within the brainstem, controls a person's state of awareness and level of consciousness. Coma following severe head injury indicates brainstem involvement and injury to the RAS. The medulla oblongata, also located within the brainstem, is the center for respiration. The cerebrum, which represents the largest mass of the brain, controls thought processes and memory, while the cerebellum controls coordination, balance, and equilibrium.

141. B. Any woman of childbearing age who has abdominal pain should be assumed to have an ectopic pregnancy until ruled out. Lower quadrant abdominal pain, especially with a history of a missed period, is a classic finding of an ectopic pregnancy. There are many causes of vaginal discharge, and tachycardia and hypotension can be the result of many other problems. Although a woman's chance of becoming pregnant is significantly higher if not on some form of birth control, many women get pregnant while on the birth control pill.

142. C. This patient, by virtue of the fact that he is conscious and screaming, clearly has a patent airway. With an isolated stab wound to the upper thigh, he does not require spinal immobilization. You must then assess what other problems may cause death. With a severed femoral artery in the upper thigh, this patient will bleed to death before you can even get your oxygen set up; therefore, bleeding should be immediately controlled.

143. D. Cystitis is an inflammation and infection of the urinary bladder and is characterized by urinary frequency (polyuria), urgency, and dysuria. Dysmenorrhea is abnormal pain during menstruation and is not associated with bladder infections.

144. B. Baroreceptors, also known as "pressure" receptors, are located within the carotid arteries and aorta. They are very sensitive to changes in arterial perfusion pressure (ie, blood pressure). When the baroreceptors sense a drop in blood pressure, they send signals via the sympathetic nervous system, resulting in the release of cate-cholamines (epinephrine and norepinephrine). Catecholamine release results in increased systemic vascular resistance (vasoconstriction) as well as increases in heart rate (positive chronotropy) and myocardial contraction force (positive inotropy).

145. C. The mechanism of and location of the injury as well as the irregularity of the patient's pulse are most suggestive of a myocardial contusion. Patients with this type of injury can experience all of the same deleterious effects associated with an acute myocardial infarction, including cardiogenic shock, arrhythmias, and cardiac arrest.

146. A. The brain, being the master organ of the body, is going to be protected by the sympathetic nervous system (SNS) at all costs. Through vasoconstriction and the shunting of blood, the catecholamines of the SNS attempt to maintain adequate cerebral perfusion.

147. B. During the initial assessment, a patient with signs suggestive of shock must receive immediate shock management. One of the easiest and most effective ways to reduce the negative effects of internal bleeding is to elevate the lower extremities 6″ to 12″, which causes blood from the lower extremities to flow towards the core of the body where the more vital organs are located. IV therapy and the inflation of the PASG (if indicated) are best performed en route to the hospital. Oxygen therapy will increase the oxygen content of the blood but will not redirect blood flow to more vital organs.

148. D. A critical incident defusing is typically performed within 2 to 4 hours after the incident and is an informal process designed to provide immediate relief and support to all who were involved in the incident. A critical incident defusing should be held no later than 12 hours after the incident. A critical incident stress debriefing (CISD) is a formal process that should occur within 24 hours but no later than 72 hours following the incident.

149. C. Diphenhydramine is an antihistamine and is indicated as a second line medica-tion to epinephrine in patients with a severe allergic reaction. The dose is 25 to 50 mg IV. In patients with severe allergic reactions (ie, anaphylaxis), intramuscular injections will not be as effective since circulation of blood through the muscles is diminished, resulting in a delayed effect of the drug. Diphenhydramine IM can be given in patients with mild to moderate allergic reactions, where the patient is not hypoperfused.

150. A. The ratio of red blood cells to plasma is called the hematocrit value. This test is used to determine the presence of internal bleeding in trauma patients. If the hematocrit is low, which indicates a greater volume of plasma, the patient is most likely bleeding internally. Likewise, if the hematocrit is elevated, plasma is being lost (ie, severe burns). The normal hematocrit value varies with the gender of the person, but on average is approximately 45%. Carboxyhemoglobin reflects the percentage of carbon monoxide that is attached to the hemoglobin molecule.

151. B. The diving reflex, also known as the mammalian diving reflex, is a protective mechanism of the body that is most prominent in cold temperatures (ie, falling in cold water). Through increased parasympathetic tone, the pulse rate and blood pressure both fall to decrease overall oxygen demand and consumption, while at the same time, blood is shunted to the brain to sustain it for as long as possible. The diving reflex is the reason why young adults and children are able to survive for extended periods of time when submerged in cold water. The effect of the diving reflex diminishes with age.

152. D. The incident commander has control over the logistical operations at the scene of a mass-casualty incident (MCI); however, the EMS medical director is ultimately responsible for all patient care-related activities. It is important that the incident commander remain in close contact with the medical director during a MCI.

153. B. Recalling that the right side of the brain controls the left side of the body and vice versa, this patient has experienced an ischemic stroke on the right side of the brain. Ischemic strokes typically present with confusion, unilateral weakness (hemiparesis), a facial droop, and dysarthria (slurred speech). The pupil is affected on the same side as the stroke because of the crossover of optic nerves within the optic chiasm in the occipital lobe of the brain. A hemorrhagic stroke typically presents with a sudden, severe headache, a rapid loss of consciousness, and signs of increased intracranial pressure (ie, hypertension, bradycardia, and respiratory abnormalities).

154. A. In addition to infectious processes, pyrogens (fever-causing agents) are also released from white blood cells in response to inflammation and act as chemical mediators on the hypothalamus. This is a normal response in both children and adults.

155. C. If you can imagine a motorcycle striking a fixed object, the operator will be ejected, striking his or her legs on the handlebars, which fractures one or both of the femurs. The operator then typically strikes the ground or object head first.

156. B. Aspirin (acetylsalicylic acid) overdoses will produce a high fever and metabolic acidosis. As the respiratory system attempts to rid the body of the excess acid and hydrogen ions, the patient's respirations will become deep and rapid. Acetaminophen overdoses result in liver damage or failure. Codeine is a narcotic and will depress the central nervous system, causing slow, shallow breathing. Ibuprofen overdoses typically result in gastrointestinal damage.

157. A. The liver is a very large, highly vascular organ that produces fibrinogen and prothrombin, both of which are essential proteins for blood clotting. In addition, the blood within the liver parenchyma does not clot. Because of these factors, lacerations of the liver are frequently the result of death because of exsanguination.

158. B. The patient's airway is rapidly swelling, as evidenced by the stridorous respirations. Additionally, his level of consciousness and vital signs are consistent with shock. After protecting the airway with an endotracheal tube, the patient should receive 0.3 to 0.5 mg (3 to 5 mL) of IV epinephrine 1:10,000.

159. D. Any condition that results in increased production or inadequate removal of bilirubin (produced by the breakdown of the hemoglobin molecule) will result in a yellowish color of the skin called jaundice. Such conditions include inflammation (hepatitis), acetaminophen overdose, and patients with chronic renal insufficiency (the kidneys do not adequately filter metabolic substrates from the blood).

160. B. The first thing that comes to mind when you think of mass-casualty incident is the word "mass," which would imply numerous patients. The fact is any situation that depletes your resources and/or ability to effectively manage the situation would be a mass-casualty incident. An example would be two critically injured patients and one ambulance. One ambulance and two medics can effectively manage one critical patient. Two critically injured patients would overwhelm them and their resources. Remember, a mass-casualty incident is not defined by patient count but rather how effectively your resources can manage the patient(s), whether they are few or many.

161. C. Arterial blood should have a high partial pressure of oxygen because it has been reoxygenated in the lungs. The normal partial pressure of arterial blood should be 80 to 100 mm Hg. An arterial PaO_2 of 60 to 80 mm Hg indicates respiratory insufficiency, while an arterial PaO_2 of less than 60 mm Hg indicates respiratory failure.

162. A. A pulse rate of less than 100 beats/min indicates hypoxia in a newborn. If the pulse rate remains below 100 beats/min after 30 seconds of assisted ventilations, the infant's airway must be checked again to ensure patency, which may include repositioning of the head to ensure a neutral position, resuctioning any secretions, or ventilating the infant with its mouth slightly open. If these techniques fail to improve the infant's respiratory status, endotracheal intubation will be needed. Chest compressions are indicated when the newborn's pulse rate falls below 60 beats/min. Dextrose should be considered if the newborn shows signs of hypoglycemia (ie, jitteriness, lethargy, pallor, etc). Naloxone should be a consideration if bradycardia and respiratory depression persist and/or if there is a history of maternal narcotic use, particularly within the previous 4 hours.

163. B. Because infants and children have a proportionately larger head when compared to an adult, this area of the body is especially vulnerable to trauma, especially from falls, in which gravity takes them head first. Deceleration incidents, where children are not properly secured or not secured at all, are also associated with head trauma. The body becomes a projectile, with the head striking the first object it encounters.

164. D. Obstructive shock results from inadequate circulation of the blood through the cardiovascular system. Injuries that can result in this type of shock include cardiac tamponade (fluid within the pericardial sac inhibits adequate contractility and decreases cardiac output), tension pneumothorax (excessive intrathoracic pressure squeezes the heart and kinks both the vena cava and aorta), and pulmonary embolism (a clot obstructs the pulmonary artery resulting in a significant strain on the right side of the heart that ultimately leads to decreased left ventricular preload and subsequent cardiac output).

165. A. When low oxygen levels are detected by the chemoreceptors in the blood, messages are sent to the diaphragm and intercostal muscles via the phrenic nerve, which originates in between the third and fifth cervical vertebrae. Injury to the cervical spine in this area can sever the phrenic nerve and result in respiratory paralysis. The chemoreceptors in the brain are located within the medulla oblongata, a part of the brainstem.

166. C. Recalling the modified Rule of Nines for children, the head accounts for 18% of the body surface area and each leg (anterior and posterior) accounts for 14%; therefore, burns to the entire head and face (18%) and anterior burns to both lower extremities (7% per leg) would total 32% of the child's body surface area.

167. B. The intravenous (IV) or intraosseous (IO) routes are clearly preferred over endotracheal (ET) drug administration for all ages. However, if IV or IO access is not available and the pediatric patient is intubated, the appropriate ET dose for epinephrine is 0.1 mL/kg (0.1 mg/kg) of a 1:1,000 solution, followed by a 5 mL flush of normal saline. IV and IO doses are given at 0.1 mL/kg (0.01 mg/kg) of a 1:10,000 solution. Higher epinephrine doses may be required if the child requires a greater adrenergic "boost" (ie, cardiac arrest caused by beta-blocker toxicity or status asthmaticus). Consult with medical control as needed.

168. C. Crystalloid solutions, such as normal saline solution and lactated Ringer's solution, will only increase the ability to circulate the red blood cells that are in the vascular space. They do not possess any oxygen-carrying capacity. Their use should not exceed 3 L in the field as they will hemodilute the blood and ultimately reduce the oxygen-carrying capacity to near zero. For every 1 mL of estimated blood loss, you should administer 3 mL of crystalloid. Colloids, such as whole blood, or synthetic substitutes such as hespan, dextran, and human plasma protein fraction contain proteins, which are larger molecules and will remain in the vascular space longer; therefore, they are replaced on 1:1 ratio for blood loss.

169. C. Critical incident stress debriefings (CISD) are a formal process that should occur as soon as possible after the incident, typically within 24 to 72 hours. The purpose of a CISD is to ensure that any issues that the providers have with regards to their inability to cope and/or feelings of guilt and severe stress are minimized as much as possible. Only the personnel directly involved in the incident participate in the CISD, which is typically mediated by counselors who specialize in this field. CISD is not intended to identify areas of weakness or lay blame on any individual, nor is it intended to serve as a method of improving one's skills.

170. B. Gases exchanged in the lungs (O_2 and CO_2) always move from an area of greater concentration to an area of lesser concentration by a process called diffusion. Blood that enters the lungs from the right side of the heart has a PO_2 of approximately 40 mm Hg and a PCO_2 of approximately 46 mm Hg. Within the lungs, carbon dioxide diffuses from the bloodstream into the alveoli while oxygen diffuses from the alveoli into the bloodstream. The partial pressure of oxygen within the alveoli is near 100 mm Hg, while the partial pressure of carbon dioxide is near 0 mm Hg.

171. B. Recalling that bradycardia is associated with severe hypoxia in the pediatric age group and is an ominous sign, a 6-month-old infant with respiratory distress, lethargy, and an SAO_2 of 82% is severely hypoxic; therefore, you should expect to see a bradycardic rhythm on the cardiac monitor, which may or may not be associated with a heart block. Idioventricular rhythms are generally not associated with a pulse, which this infant obviously has. Tachycardia in the pediatric population, as with older children and adults, is often the result of hypovolemia.

172. B. In patients with a stroke, reperfusion with fibrinolytic (thrombolytic) therapy must be initiated within 3 hours from the onset of symptoms. Additionally, patients with a history of recent major surgery (ie, hip replacement, cardiac bypass, etc) are not candidates for this therapy, nor are those with an intracranial hemorrhage or who are already taking blood-thinning medications such as warfarin. Examples of fibrinolytic medications include retivase, streptokinase, and alteplase (tPA). Fibrinolytic agents work to dissolve clots by promoting the digestion of fibrin, a key element in the blood clotting process.

173. D. Tidal volume is defined as the volume of air (in mL) that is moved in and out of the lungs in a single breath. The volume of air moved in and out of the lungs each minute is called minute volume, and is measured in liters. The average tidal volume in an average adult male is approximately 500 to 600 mL.

174. B. Nortriptyline, amyltriptyline, and clomipramine are the most commonly prescribed tricyclic antidepressant medications. Fluoxetine hydrochloride is a selective serotonin reuptake inhibitor (SSRI) that is also used to treat depression as well as obsessive-compulsive disorder. Midazolam is a benzodiazepine used for anxiolytic purposes, and buspirone is also an anxiolytic medication.

175. C. During the anger stage of the grieving process, which is typically the first stage a person enters, not only is the person angry with themselves, as in the case of a person with a terminal illness, but he or she can project that anger toward others, to include EMS personnel. It is important to understand that this displaced anger is not a personal attack on the individual to whom it is directed. All stages of the grieving process, no matter how unpleasant they can be for the patient, family, and rescuer, are healthy responses that will allow the patient or family member to come to terms with the situation.

176. C. Generalized anxiety disorder includes a broad spectrum of psychiatric problems including obsessive-compulsive disorder (OCD), panic attacks, and social phobias such as agoraphobia (fear of the market place). Schizophrenia is a severe psychiatric illness in which the patient has lost touch with reality; it is often accompanied by paranoia, hallucinations, and delusions.

177. C. The general impression is a quick formulation of the patient's condition immediately on setting your eyes on them, one of which is to assess their mental state. Patients with garbled or altered speech patterns have an altered mental state, which would clearly require more investigation.

178. A. The staging area in a mass-casualty incident is where all resources congregate and are dispatched to the most appropriate locations by the incident commander. It is at the staging area that individuals are assigned various tasks by the incident commander, such as triage officer, transport officer, and extrication officer.

179. B. Just because a patient's eyes are closed, implying that they are unconscious, does not mean that they are unconscious. The initial assessment of a patient begins by assessing the mental status. In this particular case, if it were found that the patient were unconscious, the most appropriate next step would be to move the patient to the floor and continue with the initial assessment (ie, opening the airway, assessing for breathing and pulse, etc). Since this patient was found on the couch, the chances of trauma are highly unlikely; therefore, spinal precautions would most likely not be indicated.

180. D. Because of the patient's deep and rapid respirations (may be Kussmaul respirations), a diabetic emergency is a distinct possibility. The best source for obtaining a medical history on this particular patient, in the absence of any bystanders or family members, would be to look in the patient's refrigerator where you might find insulin or the vial of life containing all of the patient's medical history and medications.

Section 3: The Paramedic Practical Examination
Answers to Dynamic Cardiology Preparatory Questions

1. List the components of the primary ABCD survey.
- **A**irway: open the airway with the head tilt-chin lift maneuver.
- **B**reathing: assess for breathing; if absent, deliver 2 breaths (1 second each).
- **C**irculation: assess for carotid pulse; if pulse is absent, begin CPR until defibrillator is present.
- **D**efibrillation: Perform quick-look with paddles or attach multi-pads to assess cardiac rhythm. If patient is in V-fib or pulseless V-tach:
  - Defibrillate one time with 360 joules followed *immediately* by CPR

2. List the components of the secondary ABCD survey.
- **A**irway: Preoxygenate the patient for 2 to 3 minutes with a BVM and then place an endotracheal tube, LMA, or dual-lumen device.
  - Confirm advanced airway placement with clinical assessment (ie, auscultation of breath sounds, adequate chest rise) *plus* another confirmation method (ie, ETCO$_2$ detector, esophageal detector device).
- **B**reathing: If patient is in cardiac arrest, ventilate at a rate of 8 to 10 breaths/min; if not in cardiac arrest, ventilate at a rate of 10 to 12 breaths/min
- **C**irculation: Assess for and manage circulation and delivery of medications:
  - Establish vascular access.
  - Attach ECG leads (unless multi-pads are used) for continuous monitoring of the cardiac rhythm.
  - Administer the appropriate medications based on the cardiac rhythm.
- **D**ifferential Diagnosis: Assess for and treat reversible causes (Hs and Ts):
  - Hypovolemia, hypoxia, hydrogen ions (acidosis), hypokalemia/hyperkalemia, hypoglycemia, hypothermia, toxins (overdose), tamponade (cardiac), tension pneumothorax, thrombosis (coronary or pulmonary), trauma (hypovolemia, increased ICP).

3. Describe your management of a patient who converts from ventricular fibrillation to sinus bradycardia **without a pulse** following defibrillation.
- Continue CPR throughout the arrest (avoid unnecessary interruptions in CPR).
- Attach ECG leads (unless multi-pads are already applied).
- Intubate and confirm proper tube placement.
- Establish vascular access.
  - Administer 1 mg of epinephrine IV/IO every 3 to 5 minutes
    - May consider 40 units of vasopressin (one-time dose) to replace the first or second dose of epinephrine.
  - Administer 1 mg of atropine IV/IO every 3 to 5 minutes.
    - Maximum dose is 3 mg.
  - Assess for and treat potentially reversible causes
    - See differential diagnosis in question #2.

4. List in the correct sequence, the appropriate steps of defibrillating a patient.
- Confirm presence of V-fib or pulseless V-tach.
- Apply conductive gel/paste to paddles (unless multi-pads are used).
- Charge defibrillator to 360 joules (monophasic) or biphasic equivalent
- Apply paddles/pads to patient's chest.
  - Sternum paddle/pad to right of upper sternum
  - Apex paddle/pad at midaxillary line lateral to left nipple
    - Apply 25 lb of pressure if paddles are used
- Ensure that you and everybody else are "Clear!"
  - Verbally **and** visually ensure this!
- If using paddles: simultaneously depress both red buttons.
- If using multi-pads: press "shock" button on defibrillator.
  - If patient does not have generalized muscle depolarization (ie, he does not jump), the defibrillator did not deliver any energy.
- Immediately begin/resume CPR and reassess cardiac rhythm in 2 minutes.

5. State the indications and correct **adult** dosages for the following medications in a **cardiac** situation:
- **Epinephrine 1:10,000**
  - Indications
    - Cardiac arrest (all rhythms)
  - Dose
    - 1 mg IV/IO every 3 to 5 min.
    - Give 2 to 2.5 the IV/IO dose if administered ET.
- **Vasopressin**
  - Indications
    - Used to replace first or second dose of epinephrine for cardiac arrest.
  - Dose
    - 40 units IV/IO, given as a one-time dose.
- **Amiodarone**[1]
  - Indications
    - V-Fib/Pulseless V-Tach
      - Dose: 300 mg IV/IO; may repeat at 150 mg once in 3 to 5 min.
    - Wide/Narrow Complex Tachycardias
      - Dose: 150 mg IV/IO over 10 min.

[1] Dilute in 20 to 30 mL of D_5W; maximum dose in **all** cases is 2.2 g per 24 hours.

- **Lidocaine**[2]
  - Indications
    - V-Fib/Pulseless V-Tach
      - Initial dose: 1 to 1.5 mg/kg IV/IO.
      - Repeat doses: 0.5 to 0.75 mg/kg every 5 to 10 minutes.
      - Maximum dose: 3 mg/kg.
    - Stable V-Tach
      - Initial dose: 0.5 to 0.75 mg/kg up to 1 to 1.5 mg/kg.
      - Repeat doses: 0.5 to 0.75 mg/kg every 5 to 10 min.
      - Maximum dose: 3 mg/kg

[2] ET dose is 2 to 4 mg/kg.

- **Atropine sulfate**
  - Indications
    - Symptomatic bradycardia
      - Dose: 0.5 mg every 3 to 5 minutes
      - Maximum dose: 3 mg
    - Asystole and Bradycardic (heart rate < 60) PEA
      - Dose: 1 mg every 3 to 5 minutes
      - Maximum dose: 3 mg

6. Describe the appropriate management for a status post cardiac arrest patient with a **perfusing** sinus tachycardia and a blood pressure of 60/40 mm Hg.
   - Reassess airway and continue ventilations as needed.
   - Consider a 250 to 500 mL normal saline bolus.
   - Dopamine
     - 2 to 20 μg/kg/min titrated to hemodynamic effect (ie, systolic BP of 90 to 100 mm Hg)
   - Continuously monitor blood pressure and airway.

7. Describe the steps to take **after** the placement of an endotracheal tube in an adult.
   - Immediately inflate distal cuff with 5 to 10 mL of air and disconnect the syringe.
   - Attach BVM to ET tube.
   - Ventilate patient and confirm proper tube placement
     - Clinical assessment (ie, auscultate breath sounds, look for adequate chest rise).
     - Additional confirmation method (ie, ETCO2 monitoring, esophageal detector device).
   - Secure tube with appropriate device.
   - Reconfirm tube placement.
   - Continue ventilations at appropriate rate
     - Apneic with pulse: 10 to 12 breaths/min
     - Pulseless and apneic: 8 to 10 breaths/min

8. Describe the appropriate management for a patient with a narrow-complex tachycardia at a rate of 180, who presents with hemodynamic compromise.
   - Ensure patent airway and give 100% oxygen.
   - Establish vascular access.
   - Give sedation if patient is conscious.
   - Synchronized cardioversion (do not delay)
     - 100, 200, 300, and 360 joules.
       - Reassess patient in between shocks.

9. What should you do after administering a medication to a cardiac arrest patient, but prior to defibrillating?
   - Circulate the medication with **effective** CPR (push hard and fast) for 2 minutes, then defibrillate if indicated.

10. How would you manage a patient in ventricular tachycardia **with a pulse**, who is hemodynamically stable?
    - Ensure patent airway and give 100% oxygen.
    - Establish vascular access.
    - Administer **one** of the following antiarrhythmics
      - Amiodarone 150 mg IV over 10 min, **or**
      - Lidocaine 0.5 to 0.75 mg/kg IV push.
    - Prepare for synchronized cardioversion.

Static Cardiology Practice Scenarios

Practice Scenario 1

- Rhythm: Monomorphic Ventricular Tachycardia
- Management: Unstable Tachycardia Algorithm
  - Ensure patent airway and give 100% oxygen.
  - Establish vascular access.
  - Consider sedation.
  - Synchronized cardioversion
    - 100, 200, 300, and 360 joules.
    - Reassess patient in between shocks.
    - Be prepared to turn synchronizer off if patient becomes pulseless.

Practice Scenario 2

- Rhythm: Third-degree AV block (complete heart block)
- Management: Symptomatic Bradycardia Algorithm
  - Ensure patent airway and give 100% oxygen.
  - Establish vascular access.
  - Immediate transcutaneous pacing (TCP)
    - Consider 0.5 mg of atropine IV as temporizing measure until TCP is initiated.
  - Consider other medications
    - Epinephrine infusion at 2 to 10 µg/min
    - Dopamine infusion at 2 to 20 µg/kg/min

Practice Scenario 3

- Rhythm: Sinus Tachycardia
- Condition: Pulseless Electrical Activity (PEA)
- Management: PEA Algorithm
  - CPR
  - Intubate and establish vascular access.
  - Epinephrine 1 mg IV push every 3 to 5 min.
    - Consider 40 units of vasopressin (one-time dose) to replace first or second dose of epinephrine.
  - Consider underlying causes (ie, Hs and Ts).
    - Consider patient's history.
      - Severe nausea, vomiting, and diarrhea for 1 week.
      - MOST likely cause is hypovolemia with possible hypokalemia.
  - Administer 20 mL/kg bolus of normal saline and reassess.

Practice Scenario 4

- Rhythm: Sinus Rhythm with one (1) PAC.
- Management: Acute Coronary Syndrome (ACS) Algorithm
  - Ensure patent airway and administer 100% oxygen
  - Give 160 to 325 mg of aspirin.
  - Establish vascular access.
  - Administer 0.4 mg of nitroglycerin (NTG) SL × 3.
    - Administer 2 to 4 mg of morphine IV if NTG does not relieve pain.
    - Repeat morphine at 2 to 8 mg in 5- to 15-minute intervals.
  - Obtain 12-lead ECG.
  - Conduct field screening to determine if patient is candidate for fibrinolytic therapy.
  - Notify medical control of 12-lead findings and fibrinolytic screening.

IV Bolus Medication Practice Scenarios

Practice Scenario 1

- Drug and dose ordered: 5 mg of diazepam (Valium)
- Concentration available: Prefilled syringe containing 20 mg/mL
- How many milliliters will you give? 0.25 mL
- Appropriate rate of administration? Slow IV/IM push
- Any special considerations? Monitor respirations, heart rate, and blood pressure; CNS depression is unlikely, but could occur.

Practice Scenario 2

- Drug and dose ordered: 300 mg of amiodarone (Cordarone)
- Concentration available: Vials containing 50 mg/mL
- How many milliliters will you give? 6 mL (50 mg/mL vials × 6 vials = 300 mg)
- Appropriate rate of administration? Rapid IV push
- Any special considerations? Dilute in 20 to 30 mL of D_5W

Practice Scenario 3

- Drug and dose ordered: 0.5 mg of atropine sulfate
- Concentration available: Prefilled syringe containing 1 mg/10 mL (0.1 mg/mL)
- How many milliliters will you give? 5 mL
- Appropriate rate of administration? Rapid IV push
- Any special considerations? *Must* give rapidly; if you administer atropine too slowly, paradoxical bradycardia may occur.

Intraosseous Infusion Practice Scenarios

Practice Scenario 1

- Fluid rate per protocol: 20 mL/kg
- Child's weight: 20 lb (9 kg)
  - 20 (weight in lb) ÷ 2.2 **or** 20 (weight in lb) ÷ 2 − 10% = 9 kg
- Total volume to be administered? 180 mL
  - 20 (mL/kg) × 9 (kg) = 180 mL

Practice Scenario 2

- Fluid amount ordered: 20 mL/kg
- Child's weight: 35 lb (16 kg)
  - 35 (weight in lb) ÷ 2.2 **or** 35 (weight in lb) ÷ 2 − 10% = 16 kg
- Total volume to be administered? 360 mL
  - 20 (mL/kg) × 16 (kg) = 320 mL

Notes

Notes

Notes

Notes

Notes

Notes

Notes

Notes

CPSIA information can be obtained at www.ICGtesting.com
Printed in the USA
BVOW05s2152071213

338336BV00008B/94/P

9 780763 755188